Stress and Relaxation

Stress and Relaxation

Application to Dentistry

By

DONALD R. MORSE, D.D.S., M.A.

Associate Professor and Director, Advanced Education
Department of Endodontology
Temple University School of Dentistry
Philadelphia, Pennsylvania

and

MERRICK L. FURST, M.A., Ph.D., M.P.H.

Associate Professor and Director, Behavioral Sciences
Department of Community Dentistry
Temple University School of Dentistry
Philadelphia, Pennsylvania

Illustrated by

Donald R. Morse, D.D.S., M.A.

With a Foreword by

Patricia Carrington, Ph.D.

Department of Psychology
Princeton University
Princeton, New Jersey

CHARLES C THOMAS • PUBLISHER
Springfield • Illinois • U.S.A.

Published and Distributed Throughout the World by

CHARLES C THOMAS • PUBLISHER
Bannerstone House
301-327 East Lawrence Avenue, Springfield, Illinois, U.S.A.

ISBN 0-398-03816-3

Library of Congress Catalog Card Number: 78-7871

With THOMAS BOOKS *careful attention is given to all details of manufacturing and design. It is the Publisher's desire to present books that are satisfactory as to their physical qualities and artistic possibilities and appropriate for their particular use.* THOMAS BOOKS *will be true to those laws of quality that assure a good name and good will.*

Printed in the United States of America
V-OO-2

Library of Congress Cataloging in Publication Data

Morse, Donald R
Stress and relaxation.

Bibliography: p.
1. Dentistry--Psychological aspects. 2. Stress (Physiology) 3. Relaxation. 4. Dentist and patient. 5. Dentists--Diseases and hygiene. I. Furst, Merrick L., joint author. II. Title.
RK53.M62 617.6′001′9 78-7871
ISBN 0-398-03816-3

to

Dr. Louis L. Dubin for teaching and motivating us in the discipline of clinical hypnosis; Dr. John Martin for his sincere cooperation in performing the many physiological tests in our several joint research projects; and our families for their extreme patience during the preparation of this manuscript.

FOREWORD

ALTHOUGH stress is a universal aspect of life, organized approaches to stress management have only recently begun to attract serious interest from the health professions. Recognized as an undesirable effect of many pathological conditions and treatment modalities, the magnitude of the effect of stress on treatment *outcome* is now beginning to be appreciated. Similarly, the effects of stress on patient compliance and the role of stress in affecting the capacity of the health service professional to operate with maximum efficiency, are becoming widely recognized.

Interest in the proper management of stress coincides with the increasing role of stress in modern life and its growing toll in terms of health. An example of this is the fact that for executives alone, one estimate has it that American industry loses between $10 billion and $20 billion annually through lost work days, hospitalization and early death caused by stress.* With society's stress index climbing and strategies to combat it proliferating, research on stress is flourishing, while some 6,000 reports a year are generated.

Prescribing tranquilizers is still the most popular approach to controlling stress, with their manufacture a multi-billion dollar industry, but non-chemical devices are rapidly gaining momentum. Increasing numbers of people are seeking out natural means of stress reduction such as relaxation or exercise techniques because there is no danger of becoming addicted to them and they further self-development.

In studying stress-control techniques, Donald Morse and Merrick Furst have taken a bold step. Assembling nuggets of information from many diverse fields, they have focused on the

**The New York Times Magazine*, November 20, 1977, p. 49.

stressors relating to dentistry and have organized and reviewed an array of coping devices to combat them. Their work has much broader implications than the management of dental stress alone, however. The research done by Morse has been of particular interest to me because my field of specialization is the westernized meditative-relaxation techniques. In this area, Don Morse has had the courage to try some exciting things. He has been the first researcher to combine meditation with hypnosis; the first to study the use of meditation for pain control (either meditation used by itself, or as a form of hypnotic induction); and has conducted a pioneering study on the differential effects of internally repeated sounds (mantras) with varying types of personalities. In this approach to stress-control he has also made imaginative use of what I have termed the "meditative mood."

Meditation, conceived of in its broadest sense, has been with us, in one form or the other, through all of recorded history. It appears to be rooted in the predilection of human beings to retreat periodically from the pressures and cares of the external world and turn inward to experience a mentally "idling" state, which possesses distinct therapeutic qualities, both of a stabilizing and pain-mitigating nature.

The meditative mood is characterized by a dreamy, drifting state of consciousness which is often accompanied by an unusual openness to experiences ordinarily obscured by active, goal-directed awareness, and by a sense of harmony with our own inner rhythms and the greater rhythms of the universe. It is an anti-anxiety state, a time when we are in control of ourselves and can establish an inner balance.

What is particularly important is that *all* of us have experienced this meditative mood at times — perhaps when we were close to nature; perhaps when we were lying in the darkness just before going to sleep; or at any other moment when a sense of tranquility and inner stillness was deeply felt. It is therefore readily available for therapeutic use.

Some people require little assistance in entering such a mood. They are fortunate enough to experience a sense of inner silence frequently enough in the course of everyday life so that it is second nature to them. This ability to establish the meditative mood at will may have a profound effect upon their lives — bringing them back periodically to an inner "center" of themselves, as though a psychological gyroscope were working to right a balance. For such people, too much outwardly focused stimulation tends automatically to be followed by a period during which the motor seems to idle as the person regains a balance between his or her inner and outer self, between the experiencing of activity and the experience of being. Perhaps such people as these do not need *formal* meditation for purposes of maintaining an optimal adjustment to life, and they may well be more stress-resistant than others.

For most of those living in modern, industrialized society, however, the pace of life is determined largely by economic considerations rather than by the rhythms of human life or natural growing things and there is a dearth of spontaneously occurring quiet inner space into which the individual can retreat for refurbishing — it is people who live under these conditions who for the most part make up our patients. It therefore becomes our responsibility to offer such people whatever inner solace we can in order to cushion the pressures they face when confronted with a stressor such as a pathological condition or a therapeutic intervention.

Beyond the immediate tension-reducing effects of the meditative mood, however, there is another service that we perform when we introduce this quieting response into a patient's life. A leisurely stroll, a prayer, or listening to the gentle patter of rain as "change of pace" are not possible for most of us in today's world, especially during working hours. Even in our leisure time we may subject ourselves to prolonged sensory bombardment from a television set rather than seek quietude. Within this context of haste and perpetual stimulation, the average human being moves from task to task with almost no time to sense his or her own self and to reaffirm the basic tenet "I exist".

It is scarcely surprising therefore that the conflicts engendered by our uncertain and stressful environment are often left unresolved and that their effects upon a human organism may accumulate until a variety of psychosomatic illnesses or behavioral disturbances emerge and a stress-prone individual is created. Although the more fortunate may not become ill from such conflicts, they will in all likelihood experience a sense of meaninglessness or unease about their lives — they will have lost touch with the core of their beings.

It is within the context of this vacuum within our society that the new meditative techniques have gained their popularity. The widespread use of commercially available forms of meditation (and more recently of clinically based forms such as Benson's technique or CSM*) undoubtedly reflect a hunger on the part of Westerners for the meditative mood. Not being supplied this kind of inner refurbishing by other modalities in our society, many people are now turning to formal meditation as a means for attaining it.

This has resulted in enough solid research on the meditative-relaxation techniques so that the question to be answered is no longer whether meditative relaxation works to alleviate stress (it often does), but rather for *whom* it works and under what circumstances. We must also ask *which* meditative-relaxation technique is more beneficial for a particular individual. It is to these questions that those conducting research on the meditative-relaxation techniques are now addressing themselves.

Within this important area of inquiry, the present book assumes a unique place. Morse and Furst have drawn together a mass of data and related it to a therapeutic goal which has meaning for all of us — the greater humanization of patient care. The authors clearly do not see the patient as a person to be tranquilized or made to comply with treatment for the sake of convenience or expediency (although our own needs as human beings as well as professional persons are recognized as important parts of the therapeutic equation). Instead they see him or her as a person entitled to a meaningful therapeutic experience which is not only pain-free, but which can actually

*Benson's technique is a simple form of breathing meditation; CSM or Clinical Standardized Meditation is a westernized form of mantra meditation taught by the use of tapes and a programmed instruction text.

be rewarding and lead to increased growth and self-confidence.

Such an approach is a new way of looking at the treatment of patients. It is both democratic and positive in emphasis and it is introduced thoroughly and provocatively in the present book, with the authors actually breaking ground. It is important for us to absorb their well-stated message. By so doing, we may be able to reach a more satisfying view of our own healing roles and realize how we can provide for the full growth of our patients on all levels. In widening our perspective in this manner we can then partake of a new era in health care delivery — an era in which the humanistic management of stress emerges as a major concern and a primary goal.

Patricia Carrington, Ph.D.
Department of Psychology
Princeton University
April 7, 1978

PREFACE

THIS book is designed for two audiences: (1) dental students who are taking a course in behavioral science, psychology, or pain and anxiety control; and (2) dentists who are either in clinical practice or teaching.

The material is presented in logical order, with a thorough discussion of stress before methods of coping with stress are considered. However, for the dentist who is primarily interested in dealing with the stress of dentistry — and is well aware of what stress means — Chapters 5 and 6 may be read first.

The book is written in a nonfiction style. In order not to interrupt the flow of the narrative, the references in the body of the text have been kept to a minimum. Where there are research findings or anecdotes that amplify the discussion, they are placed in separate boxes. Some readers may choose to read the complete section first for continuity and then return to the boxes for further clarification. Other readers who desire immediate documentation may read the boxes as they come up in the text. On occasion, humorous anecdotes or illustrations have been included. These lighten the reading load, which is fairly technical at times, and they reduce the stress of the individual who may be taxed by reading a book on stress.

For those who are interested in the many sources for this book, a reference section has been included at the end of each chapter. It is sincerely hoped that this is helpful to the reader.

D.R.M.
M.L.F.

INTRODUCTION

DESPITE the rapid improvements in clinical techniques, office decor, patient management, and public education, there are still too many people who fear dental treatments. These fears keep potential patients away from the dental office and result in others arriving reluctantly and in distress.

Recent press releases and dental articles have brought to the attention of laymen and dentists alike that the practice of dentistry can induce stress-related diseases and disorders. Although the stress of dentistry has many sources, one of the major causes of dentist stress is patient stress. Continually dealing with fearful patients can result in distress to the dentist. In this book, both patient and dentist stress is covered, and means of coping with these stresses are presented.

As a preliminary to the discussion of the stress of dentistry, a thorough and clear presentation is made of the concepts of stress and relaxation. A consideration of the causes and potential cures of patients' dental fears follows. Included in the discussion are methods of pain and fear control, such as (1) behavior modification, (2) hypnosis, (3) meditation, (4) conscious sedation techniques, (5) drug therapy, (6) anesthetic methods, (7) office atmosphere, and (8) patient education. Examined next are the stress-related oral conditions, such as bruxism and the myofascial pain-dysfunction syndrome.

With respect to the dentist, an evaluation is made of stress-related diseases and disorders and how they can be managed. For the control of stress, attention is given to four major approaches: (1) the relaxation methods of hypnosis and meditation, (2) use of cardiovascular enhancing exercises, (3) nutritional supplementation, and (4) psychological coping methods. Other stress-control methods considered include diversion, consultation, and negative coping methods, e.g.

smoking, drinking, and drug use.

It is hoped that the reading of this book results in a better understanding of the stressors of dentistry. Furthermore, practicing the coping methods as outlined should lead to greater acceptance of dentistry by patients and greater enjoyment of practice by dentists. The ultimate goal is "success without distress."

D.R.M.
M.L.F.

ACKNOWLEDGMENTS

THE material necessary to write this textbook was gathered from a variety of sources, including clinical practice, research studies, personal experience, and review of the literature. In those various avenues, we had help continually. Therefore, we would like to thank the following people for their support:

Mr. Alex V. Mucha, Director of Visual Education, Temple University School of Dentistry, for the excellence of the photographic reproductions.

Mr. Andrew Morse and Mr. Brian Morse, photographers, Cherry Hill, New Jersey, for their help in the photography.

Dr. Robert (Rufus) Minor, third-year resident, Department of Endodontology, Temple University School of Dentistry, for Figure 5-1.

The Endodontology graduate students, for their thoughtful suggestions.

Dr. Samuel Seltzer, Professor and Chairman, Department of Endodontology, Temple University School of Dentistry, for his helpful suggestions and continued encouragement.

Ms. Virginia Lampson and the dental school library staff, for helping us find the many periodicals and books we required.

Dr. Gerald Orner, Associate Professor and Chairman, Department of Community Dentistry, Temple University School of Dentistry, for his continued support.

Mr. Jed Margolis and Mrs. Diane F. Morse, physical education teachers, Cherry Hill, New Jersey, for their contributions to the exercise section in Chapter 6.

Dr. Norma Furst, Dean of Student Affairs, Temple University, for reading and helping in the editing of the manuscript.

Mr. Payne Thomas and the staff of Charles C Thomas, Publisher, for their sincere cooperation in the publication of this text.

Dr. Richard Mumma, Acting Dean, New York University College of Dentistry, for his inspiration and encouragement.

Dr. Martin Tansy, Professor and Chairman, Department of Biophysics and Physiology, Temple University, for his cooperation in the use of facilities and staff for our several joint research projects.

D.R.M.
M.L.F.

CONTENTS

Stress and Relaxation

CHAPTER 1

STRESS AND RELAXATION

Stress is examined biochemically, physiologically, pathologically, and psychologically in commonsense terms. The stress concept is divided into stressors, the individual's make-up, and the actual changes. The differences between stress, neustress, eustress, and distress are considered. Also differentiated are pressure, tension, and anxiety. Relaxation is examined on the same dimensions as stress. The differences between physical and mental relaxation are reviewed.

STRESS

Introduction

YOU glance at your watch. It is 4:05 PM. The front doorbell chimes. (That must be the four o'clock patient.) As you stare at the third rubber-base impression, it still shows that you've missed the distal margin. "Sorry, Mrs. Francona, we'll have to retake that impression." (If that darn lab didn't mess up the casting, the crown would be in by now.) And the little brat, Jimmy, is crying in the second treatment room. In comes Mildred, "Dr. Pierce, it's your wife on the phone. She said that Bobby wrecked the Olds." Meanwhile, Karen loads the tray. Your head is pounding, but you count to ten; your hands are shaking, but you grab the tray. You start to take the impression and . . . Mrs. Francona sneezes, Jimmy screams, Karen faints, the rubbery goo smears your hands and sleeves and the radio announcer calmly states, "The Dow Jones Industrial Average dropped another ten points today to reach a yearly low of . . . "

No one has to define your internal state — You are under stress. But what do we really know about stress?

Over forty years ago, Hans Selye published his first paper on *biologic stress*. Since then, there have been over 110,000 publications related to stress. Yet, there is great confusion over the meaning and significance of biologic stress. In physics, *stress* is defined as a force applied per unit area to an object. *Strain* is the deformation of the object as a result of the applied stress: The external stress induces the internal strain. However, in biology, both the external forces and the internal changes have been labeled as *stress*. For example, one reads about mental and physical stresses that are analogous to the external stress of physics. But Selye's concept of stress is the nonspecific response of the body, which is analogous to the internal strain of physics. Although we believe that the biologic use of these terms should follow the physics usage, because of their popularity, Selye's terms are used with slight modifications.

Stressors

In this book, the terms *stressful stimuli* or *stressors* are designated for external stress. Hence, stressors are any physical, social, or psychological factors, events, or conditions that have the potentiality to induce certain physiological and psychological changes in a given individual at a particular time. Collectively, the changes are known as *stress* or the *stress response*. Stress is necessary for the day-to-day adaptability of man to his environment (homeostasis.) The strength, duration, and timing of the stressor and the specific makeup of the individual determine how he reacts to the stressor to produce a particular stress response. If the response is necessary for adaptability but is essentially neutral in effect, it is known as *neustress*. If the response is favorable and results in an improvement in health (Box 1-1), it is designated as *eustress*. (The prefix *eu* denotes good or healthy, as in the word *eugenics*.) If the response is unfavorable and potentially disease producing, it is called *distress*. However, there is overlap with these responses, and the designations only indicate general trends. In Figure 1-1, the interrelationship of stressors and stress is shown in simplified form.

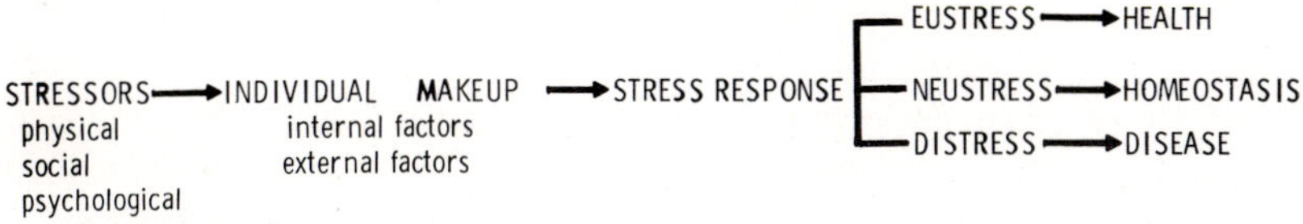

Figure 1-1. The interrelationship of stressors, stress, and clinical states.

Box 1-1: Sound Mind Sound Body

By definition, *health* is not merely the absence of disease. An individual can have a pulse rate of 95 and a blood pressure reading of 140/90 and have no symptoms or signs of disease and be considered "normal." Yet, with all other considerations being equal, a person with a pulse rate of 60 and a blood pressure reading of 110/65 would be considered in a better state of health than the individual who was described previously. There is evidence that regular, progressive exercise that involves a series of stress reactions can promote beneficial physiological changes that can prevent such conditions as cardiovascular diseases. It also appears that a positive mental attitude is important to promote psychological health. For example, rather than react to a stressor with anger, one could react with a smile. Selye (1974) says that we should react positively in order to "earn our neighbor's love."

The following are possible stressors.

Physical Stressors

Physical stressors are externally induced and include factors such as trauma, chemicals, drugs, foods, infection, hot, cold, noise, radiation, and exercise. Host resistance modifies the response, but if the agents are sufficiently intense and enduring, they produce distress in any individual.

Social Stressors

Social stressors are also externally induced and result from the interaction of the individual with his environment. They often are unforeseen and traumatic and include such occurrences as death of a loved one, divorce, loss or change in a job, and forced relocation. Pleasant events, such as engagements and marriages, can also be social stressors. Stoical individuals outwardly appear to react favorably to negative social stressors, but they may be "churning" inwardly. However, if the stressor is severe enough, e.g. death of a spouse, almost everyone reacts with distress.

Psychological Stressors

Psychological stressors may be externally induced by physical or social stressors, or they may be internally induced. Psychological stressors include anger, frustration, guilt, disgust, worry, hate, love, happiness, sadness, fear, feelings of inferiority, and anxiety. Except for anxiety, the others are brought on by physical or social stressors or the mental review of those stressors. For example, in the introduction to this chapter, the problems with the dental impressions, the screaming child, the doorbell chiming, and telephone interruptions were all physical stressors that caused the dentist to become angry and frustrated (psychological stressors).

Frustration occurs when an individual is blocked from achieving a goal and feels annoyed, confused, or angry as a result. Often, the frustration comes not only from a single obstacle but from a conflict of two important needs or goals in which choosing either alternative means frustration in regard to the other. Neal Miller (1959) has conveniently classified these conflicts into the following three categories:

1. In *approach-avoidance* conflicts, there are strong tendencies to both approach and to avoid the same goal. As an example, a dental student strives towards the D.D.S. degree, and simultaneously he cuts classes because of lack of interest in basic science subject matter.

2. In *double-approach* conflicts, there is competition between two or more desirable goals. For example, a college student

may have to choose between going to dental or medical school.

3. In *double-avoidant* conflicts, there are strong tendencies to avoid both goals. Consider the plight of the dental student who feels guilty because he cheated on an exam but at the same time is fearful of being caught.

Feelings of inferiority (Box 1-2) can be brought on by legitimate physical stressors, e.g. being very short, obese, or physically disfigured.

Box 1-2: Little Giants and Giant Little People

Compensation is a strenuous effort to make up for failure or weakness in one activity through excelling in either a different or an allied activity. According to Alfred Adler, one of the early psychoanalysts who broke with Sigmund Freud, a peculiar form of compensation, *overcompensation,* is an attempt to deny a weakness by trying to excel where one is weakest. The weakness thus acts as a goad to superior performance.

Napoleon, who was of short stature, may have suffered a sense of powerlessness for which he overcompensated by a struggle for political might. Thus, if someone uses an energetic and effective (though not necessarily admirable) method of meeting weakness, his stress response may be more of a eustress type. In contradistinction, if excessive emotion accompanies the stress response, the individual may develop an inferiority complex, and the stress response may be more of a distress type (Adler, 1917).

Anxiety is usually an internally induced stressor. It is related to an irrational fear that may be brought on by some external occurrence. More often, it is based on a person's subjective, distorted view of a situation. For example, the individual who panics at the thought of going to the dentist even though he has never had dental treatment would be suffering from dental anxiety. Anxiety provokes distress; distress leads to added anxiety.

The effects of physical and social stressors are based to a large degree on the strength and duration of the involved stressor. However, with psychological stressors, the results are intimately associated with how the individual interprets and reacts to the particular stressor. For example, a person placed in a dental chair and faced with a dentist, a drill and no novocaine would become seriously alarmed. Undoubtedly, his fear would be intense and related to the strong possibility that he would soon be in extreme pain. This situation would result in a state of distress. Yet, the alarm could be stilled by an expert in self-hypnosis who could obtain deep analgesia. Thus, the resultant reaction might be neustress or even eustress, if the self-hypnotic state was perceived as pleasant.

Even though host resistance is important with psychological stressors, if the situation creates intense emotion, expecially if prolonged, then distress results. Fear of the unknown is a severe psychological stressor that usually yields distress. A more concrete example occurs with soldiers in combat (Box 1-3).

Box 1-3: Battle Fatigue

The combination of physical stressors, e.g. fighting an unseen enemy for days and weeks and the intense anxiety experienced from not knowing whether or not survival is possible, can cause "normal" soldiers to behave abnormally. This behavior is known as *battle fatigue*. Interestingly enough, some individuals who cope well with difficult problems in civilian life may still suffer battle fatigue under the unusually stressful combat situation. Other individuals may even suffer "battle fatigue" under the ordinary difficulties of everyday life.

Physics-related Terms

Certain physics-related terms have been used as synonyms for stress, but they really are examples of psychological or physical stressors. One such term is *tension*. The physicist's *tension* is a force tending to produce extension or elongation. *Nervous tension* and *mental tension* are pseudobiological terms referring to feelings of uneasiness and anxiety. The person feels "keyed-up" or "stressed." *Muscle tension* usually refers to being "tensed-up" or "uptight." It is presumed that the body's muscles are in a state of extreme contraction and are "coiled for action," but no external action takes place to relieve the tension. *Muscle tension* has also been used synonymously with *nervous tension.* True muscle tension refers to the partial contraction of the supporting muscles of the body that maintain a state of muscle tonus. Muscle tension can also occur in other muscle groups as the result of psychological stressors such as anger, frustration, worry, and anxiety. The partial contraction constricts blood vessels and causes nerve fibers to become hypersensitive. The end result is pain. The most common painful conditions that occur are tension headache, myofascial pain, shoulder pain, and backache. These conditions can be treated by muscle reconditioning through exercise and deep muscular relaxation (*see* Chaps. 5 and 6).

Pressure is another term borrowed from the physical science vocabulary that is used erroneously as a synonym for stress. In physics, *pressure* refers to the force applied per unit area of a surface. The familiar phrase "the pressures of society" refers to the psychosocial stressors of everyday life.

Individual Makeup

Introduction

The makeup of the individual consists of those mediating and conditioning factors that are primarily responsible for how the stress response appears. Is it eustress, neustress or distress? (Box 1-4)

Box 1-4: Stress Now and Then

Stress is a normal, important response. Without it, people could not survive. For example, if you were driving and another car suddenly came toward you at full speed, you would live to tell the story only if you had immediately swerved your car and thereby produced stress. Had you chosen to respond by sitting behind the wheel and meditating, you might have temporarily achieved eustress, but you would have ended up by being the most peaceful soul in the grave. Hence, it can be seen that the normal stress response is essential. (Some degree of stress results from just breathing, walking, or talking.) However, there are not many situations in today's life-style in which an extreme stress response is called for (as indicated by the car story).

With primitive man, who had to fight or flee for survival, extreme stress responses were important. In contemporary society, quite often when we are in stress-provoking situations, we neither fight nor run. Instead, we become angry, afraid, tense, rigid, or "freeze." These reactions can lead to distress and eventual disease, especially if the stressful situations are repeated. Still, some people can cope without being distressed.

The various responses result from differences in the individual makeup, which is determined by internal and external factors.

Internal Factors

Internal factors are based on the individual's genetic constitution and environmental modifications. This leads to the concept of stress tolerance or *safety zone*. If the threshhold of an individual's stress tolerance is exceeded, then distress can result. The various internal factors include the following:

1. Certain individuals are genetically programmed to respond to stressors with an excessive sympathetic nervous system response. These people are called *sympathicotonics*. They are prone to develop severe stress responses as a result of an outpouring of catecholamines. Other individuals respond with an excessive parasympathetic response. They are known as *vagotonics* and their severe stress response is related to acetylcholine release.

2. There are rare individuals that are apparently born without the ability to perceive pain and other external stimuli (congenital dysautonomia). Ernest Hilgard (1975) has described people who receive severe physical stressors such as burns, cuts, and trauma and yet do not react nor subjectively report painful sensations. Although this sounds as if it might be an advantage, that is not the case because these people may suffer severe

inflammatory and degenerating diseases without the warning benefit of pain.

3. Stressors can also occur without any conscious perception. For example, cancer may be far advanced before any clinical manifestations become apparent.

4. About 15 percent of the population are *allergic* individuals. They respond to certain external stressors, such as pollen, dust, and bacteria with parasympathetic responses. For example, asthmatics produce acetylcholine, which results in bronchial constriction.

5. In the normal development of an individual, certain major changes occur during which the person may be more susceptible to stressors. These are related to genetically induced periods that can be greatly influenced by the environment. For example, the teenage years are more stressful than the ages from seven to ten. Jean Piaget (1954) described childhood development, and the *psychosocial crises* of Erik Erikson (1950) and the *passages* (predictable crises) of Gail Sheehy (1976) delineate adult development. At times of normal life changes, distress and disease may result.

6. Unsuccessful attempts have been made to correlate human body morphology, e.g. ectomorph (lean), endomorph (corpulant), and mesomorph (muscular), with the ability to cope with stressors (Sheldon, 1954).

7. There are many so-called personality types, and individuals of each type can react differently to stressors.

a. The earliest attempt at personality typing was by Carl Jung (1923) — a contemporary of Freud — who classified people into *introverts* and *extroverts.* The introvert, especially in time of emotional stress or conflict, tends to withdraw into himself and "seethe" internally. The extrovert, by contrast, when under stress, tends to lose himself among people and by "blowing off steam" may relieve stress.

b. According to Julian Rotter (1966), people can also be regarded as *externals* or *internals.* Individuals can be identified through a measure of personality called *locus of control.* Briefly, locus of control is a belief held by people regarding the degree to which they consider themselves as being in control of whatever happens to them. The "internal" believes that he is in control of what happens, whereas the "external" believes that whatever happens to him is a result of luck, fate, or "superior beings." In the extreme form, the external orientation is paranoia.

c. In simple language, people can also be regarded as *uppers* and *downers.* Such individuals are characterized by mood swings in the direction either of excitement and elation or of fatigue, despondency, and sadness. During the "up" phase, stress situations are perceived positively and managed well. During the "down" phase, the reverse is true. In its extreme form, the cycle (cyclothymic) is classified as a *manic-depressive reaction.*

d. There are people who avoid situations in which they may be required to compete. While personality disorganization may not be apparent, in its extreme form this is classified as *schizophrenia.*

e. The *explosive* or *aggressive* personality tends to lose control when he is frustrated and is confronted with some minor stressors. This negative reaction may be an extreme behavior of the extrovert discussed earlier.

f. The *obsessive-compulsive* individual pays excessive attention to petty details. There is a lack of tolerance for stressors, and conflicts are avoided by strict adherence to rules and conventions; changes or deviations from accustomed routines are upsetting. The insistence on perfection may be descriptive of the obsessive-compulsive dentist.

g. The *hysterical* personality may have masochistic needs for experiencing suffering or pain on an unconscious level. Perhaps such individuals enjoy their hypochondria and are forever seeking physical problems even when negative results are forthcoming from diagnostic medical tests.

h. Negativistic people tend to be *passive-aggressive.* In their opposition they do not express open aggression and refuse to face stressors. In its extreme form, ignoring or avoiding stressors can lead to depression.

i. The *passive-dependent* person is shy, submissive, and dejected. Such an individual does not voice an opinion, is afraid to offend, does not exercise independent judgement, and suppresses emotion. As a result, such an individual copes poorly and tends to have many physical ailments. In an extreme form, this person suffers hypochondria (*see* g above).

j. The *antisocial* or *sociopathic* personality gratifies impulses and egocentric desires. These individuals tend to lie, blame others, and are prone to using defense mechanisms. There is a low frustration tolerance and a tendency to discharge their stress by harming others. In its extreme form, such people are classified as *psychopathic*.

k. The *asthenic* or detached, passive, asocial personality, has a low energy level, is easily fatigued by physical stressors, and is marked by an absence of zest for living.

l. The *dependent-passive, submissive,* or *inadequate* personality is not mentally deficient, although at times he or she may appear stupid. Such an individual does not appear to do anything correctly, is inept, and gives ineffectual responses. In its extreme form, the frustrations may lead to schizophrenia.

m. The "spoiled-child" reaction may be found in the *narcissistic* personality. Such an individual tends to be egocentric, disdainful, boastful, and may appear self-assured. His mere desire is sufficient justification for what he seeks; others are expected to subordinate their desires to his comfort.

n. Personalities are also classified into *Type A* or *Type B*. These types are related to susceptibility to coronary artery disease and are discussed in Chapter 4.

8. Psychoanalysts classify according to *character disorders,* which overlaps several of the personality descriptions given above, e.g. oral, anal, urethral, and phallic.

9. Normal individuals also appear to have *cyclic changes* related to emotional state, hormonal and enzymatic activity, weather, time of day, atmospheric ions, season, geographic location, genetic background, and astrological signs (according to some believers). These changing cycles are known as *biorhythms*. During so-called bad periods, people might respond negatively to stressors and vice versa. There seems to be a sex difference in that females appear to react worse to stressors just before and during the menses, as compared to other days of the month (premenstrual tension). After

menopause, females who previously were resistant then become just as prone as males to stress-related diseases, e.g. hypertension. Hormonal changes are probably responsible for the latter two findings.

10. There are some individuals who actively seek certain stressors that per se might not be pleasurable, in order to experience the exhilaration received from the relief of that stress (Box 1-5).

11. There is recent evidence that the hemispheres of the brain are specialized with respect to the manner in which they process information (Samples, 1975).

Box 1-5: The "Rush"

According to R. L. Solomon (1956), many parachute jumpers, for example, engage in that type of activity for the "rush" experienced upon landing safely. The jump is life threatening, and the relief is the escape or return from death. Similarly, soldiers anticipate the stress of battle not necessarily because they enjoy it, but because of the release of stress that may be obtained from the actual fight or the realization that they survived the battle.

Consider the person who either beats himself or gets beaten (a form of masochism). He may tolerate it for the same reason. "Keep beating me; it feels good when you stop."

Some people take drugs, alcohol, or tobacco in increasing amounts for the "high" received later, even though they know that they are damaging themselves and it is a slow form of suicide. They may even dislike the taste of the drug, e.g. Scotch, but persist in order to get the subsequent enjoyment.

There are actually some patients who go to the dentist expecting to be hurt and who want to feel pain. Again, it may be the relief from the pain afterwards that is being sought. For example, Borland (1962) observed dental patients who reported enjoying painful dental treatment. "One of these was a woman who insisted upon having her teeth removed without anesthesia, and gave every indication of a kind of detached ecstasy in the face of what must have been excruciating pain."

In a right-handed individual, the left hemisphere processes analytical, logical, and verbal information (*rational type*) whereas the right hemisphere processes gestalt, holistic, and spacial information (*emotional type*). In Western societies, emphasis is placed on left brain activity; in Eastern societies, right brain activity is emphasized. Apparently, Eastern yogis handle stress well, and it may be important to train individuals to increase right brain activity. There also may be some genetic influence on the relative use of left and right cerebral hemispheres.

12. *Age* is an internal factor affecting susceptibility to stress. Young children often react well to the potential stressors of the dental office. Yet, if a child is threatened by his mother about being taken to the dentist, then the first dental visit will be anxiety provoking. Older individuals have a poorer resistance to infection and apparently a lower tolerance to stressful situations. This is compounded if they have had previous negative experiences. Consider the patient who becomes so sensitized by previous painful dental visits and "horror stories" from others that he arrives in the reception room in a state of panic.

13. *Sex* is another internal factor. Women's hormonal variation has already been discussed. When faced with stressful situations, men are more prone to become angry, as they have been socialized to not show fear. Rather than become angry, women are more likely to become anxious and cry. Anger is often only an illusion of strength. The harmful distress method of anger substitutes for beneficial fighting and crying.

14. *Ethnic origin* is another internal consideration. People of different races, religions, and nationalities may react differently to certain stressors. The influences are based on a combination of genetic and environmental factors: (a) When painful stimuli are presented to different ethnic groups, studies have shown that reactions are quicker among Jews, Italians, and Frenchmen, as compared to Orientals, Yankees (Old Americans), and Scandinavians (Hilgard and Hilgard, 1975; Seltzer, 1971); (b) Certain diseases are primarily genetic but may be precipitated by stressful incidents occurring in different ethnic groups. These include diabetes and Gaucher's disease in Jews,

Cooley's anemia in Italians and Greeks, and sickle cell anemia in blacks (Morse, 1974).

External Factors

External factors affecting the individual's makeup include disease, fatigue, diet, drug intake, occupation, location, family structure, physical fitness, mental functioning, and the ability to relax. Although disease, diet, and drugs are physical stressors in themselves, these factors can also affect individuals such that they have altered responses to other stressors. The many external factors include the following:

1. Actual or even subclinical disease states can affect how a person responds to stressors. For example, people with immunological diseases — Addison's disease (deficiency of corticoid production) or Cushing's disease (overabundance of corticoid production) — or who are on immunosuppressant drugs, such as cortisone, often have poor stress responses. Moreover, the presence of mental diseases, e.g. schizophrenia, or the treatment of these diseases, e.g. drugs, shock treatment, or prefrontal lobotomy, can greatly affect how an individual responds to stressors. When an individual is fatigued (either physically or mentally), his ability to cope with stressors is greatly diminished.

2. Although all the evidence is not available, it does appear that inadequate diets can contribute to poor resistance to stressors and that vitamin and mineral supplements can enhance one's ability to counteract stressors. Of special interest as antistress vitamins are the B complex group and vitamin C (*see* Chap. 6).

3. Various drugs can affect resistance to stressors. For example, excessive alcohol intake decreases the body's immune response. This, in turn, could cause inadequate coping responses to microbial or viral infections (Morse, 1974).

4. Undoubtedly, a person's occupation has a great deal to do with the number and type of stressors to which he is subject and how he reacts to them. Psychiatrists, dentists, and business executives are in stressful occupations.

5. Whether one practices or lives in the city, country, or suburbs has an important effect on stress levels. There are undoubtedly more stressors associated with city living, as compared to the others.

6. The family situation is related to stress. The stability of the marriage, in-law problems, presence or absence of children, whether single or divorced, whether living at home or away from home; all of these factors affect stressors and the stress response.

7. If one is physically prepared, he would be better able to cope with physical stressors. For example, a weight lifter could pick up 200 pounds over his head and react with a beneficial eustress response. An overweight, sedentary dentist attempting that same feat might react with a severe distress reaction that could precipitate a coronary occlusion. There is some evidence that mental training can also help in the management of physical stressors (Box 1-6).

Box 1-6: "Toughening-Up"

Neal Miller (1977a and b) did an interesting experiment with rats. Previous experiments had shown that when rats were exposed to shocks they developed a significantly higher incidence of stomach ulcers and corticosteroid levels than rats not so exposed. The rats also had significantly poorer subsequent learning ability than unshocked rats.

In the current experiment, the A group of rats were exposed to shocks for fifteen consecutive days. On the sixteenth day, the rats received additional shocks. The B group received the shocks only on the sixteenth day. The "toughened-up" rats (A group) had significantly less ulcers and corticosteroid levels than the untrained B group. The A group also had better subsequent learning performances than the B group.

In a follow-up experiment, it was found that when shocks were repeated at closer intervals (than daily as in the previous experiment), then those rats did worse than any of the other groups. So, with training for stress coping, it appears that there must be a sufficient time interval for adaptability.

In a primitive society, if you were challenged by someone, you could fight and there would be a beneficial release during the stress response (that is, if you survived without serious injury). In today's Western society, when challenged or punched, you might think twice about fighting back. Instead, you would probably "churn" inside, possibly resort to a lawsuit, and let the stress response stay internal. No beneficial release from muscular activity would occur, and hypertension or an ulcer could be the eventual result.

With warring tribes of the long past and during revival meetings, chanting and shouting often occurred. As with actual fighting, vocal release is beneficial. In this connection, primal scream therapy is discussed in Chapter 6.

8. Strong positive attitudes enable one to cope better with stressors, whereas negative attitudes can lead to distress and disease (*see* Chap. 4). Mental preparedness is also important. Consider the following. If you were to face a large audience and were asked to lecture on the treatment of dental caries, you would probably not overreact with fear if you were well versed on that subject. But if you had to talk on a subject not within your training, such as immunology, panic might set in.

Knowledge can change possible distress to eustress. For example, a harmless water snake in the path of an ordinary individual often provokes a serious distress reaction. While in trance, a yogi would probably go on meditating as the snake writhed under his feet.

9. Emotional stability and the ability to relax are also key factors in the management of stressors. A positive outlook can change a potentially distressful situation into eustress. Being calm in the face of adversity, giving praise instead of negative criticism, smiling instead of frowning, channelling work into productive outlets; all of these can satisfy one's ego, "earn one's neighbor's love," and as a bonus, promote psychological health. Being slightly apprehensive can also be effective at times. Before a lecture or an athletic contest, psyching up and the flow of adrenaline often allow for a better performance.

The Stress Response

After stressors and the individual's makeup, the physiological and psychological characteristics of the stress response are examined. Whether the stressor is local, a burned hand, or general, being thrown into an ice-cold bath, there is a rather specific stress response generated. Aside from this stress response, there are other physiologic responses that occur that are related to the particular stressor. For example, with the burned hand, there is an inflammatory response with the release of histamine, plasma kinins, and lysosomal enzymes. Aside from the particular response, there is the overriding stress response. The stress response begins with some internal message. This message is carried by the first mediator to the hypothalamus. The nature of the first mediator is not definitely known, but there is some evidence that it is one of the prostaglandins (small chemical substances involved in inflammation). However, physical damage is not necessary for the initiation of the stress response. Precursors of the catecholamines may also be involved in the first mediation.

Once the hypothalamus is alerted, two primary systems become activated. The first is the hypothalamus-anterior pituitary-adrenal cortex (H-AP-AC) axis, which results in the release of corticosteroids. The second is the autonomic nervous system response with the primary release of epinephrine and norepinephrine (catecholamines).

Part of the evidence showing that these systems are involved in stress has been gathered from experiments in which there was either electrical stimulation of a part of the hypothalamus or systemic injections of corticosteroids and catecholamines (Benson, 1974; Kopin, 1976; Selye, 1976b).

Hypothalamus-Anterior Pituitary-Adrenal Cortex Axis

With the H-AP-AC system, the hypothalamus releases into the blood stream a corticotropin releasing factor (CRF), which induces the anterior pituitary gland (adenohypophysis) to produce adrenocorticotropic hormone (ACTH) (Box 1-7). ACTH then travels in the blood stream to the adrenal cortex, which responds by releasing the syntoxic steroids (glucocorticoids, or anti-inflammatory corticoids such as cortisone). At the same time, but to a lesser degree, the anterior pituitary releases another hormone into the blood stream, somatotropin (STH or growth hormone). STH then travels to the adrenal cortex and apparently induces the release of catatoxic steroids (mineralocorticoids, or pro-inflammatory corticoids, such as aldosterone). These two groups of steroid hormones (syn- and catatoxic) act in harmony during the normal stress response, with the result being the maintenance of the internal environment. However, with distress, there is apparently excess syntoxic steroid production, and dangerous levels may build up. During a neutral state, corticoid excess signals ACTH to cut off production, which tones down the reaction. This feedback response does not work during stress, and excess corticoids can accumulate, especially if the reaction becomes chronic. Some of the results of corticoid action are now examined.

Box 1-7: Stress, the Superprotein, and the Cyclics

Recent research by Udenfriend resulted in the identification of a large protein, *pro-opiocortin,* that is supposedly released from the anterior pituitary in times of acute stress. Soon after release this molecule breaks up into smaller pieces: endorphins and enkephalins, MSH (melanocyte-stimulating hormone), and ACTH. Each of these smaller molecules then is directed to its own target tissue. ACTH acts on the adrenal cortex, and the end result is the release of corticosteroids. The endorphins and enkephalins are endogenous morphinelike substances that are apparently useful in controlling stress-related pain. The release of endorphins and enkephalins may account for the well-known phenomenon that pain is decreased during emergency situations, such as in military combat. The role of MSH in stress is not known (Beecher, 1956; Leff, 1978).

With all hormone action, including ACTH, there is a second messenger system that acts at the cell membrane and activates the enzyme that induces the release of the secondary substance. This second messenger system is the *cyclic nucleotides,* specifically cyclic AMP (adenosine 3′: 5′-monophosphate) and cyclic GMP (guanosine 3′:5′-monophosphate.) Recent evidence has shown that ACTH primarily induces the activation of cyclic GMP at the adrenal cortex, which then activates a protein kinase that causes the release of corticosteroids (Perchellet, 1978).

Cortisone inhibits inflammation. It inactivates lymphoid tissue (thymus and lymph nodes), lymphocytes, polymorphonuclear leucocytes, and macrophages. This allows infections to spread. Cortisone stimulates glucose production (gluconeogenesis). During a normal stress reaction, this is important, since glucose supplies energy needed for muscular work, e.g. fighting an enemy or running away from a fire. Unfortunately, excess production of glucose in a susceptible individual could lead to the development of diabetes.

Corticoids also act in the bronchioles of the lungs, causing dilation. This apparently aids in the stress response by allowing for a better exchange of respiratory gases. Excess cortisone irritates the lining of the digestive tract and leads to the development of peptic ulcers (Box 1-8).

Box 1-8: The Ulcer-Prone Rat

Neal Miller (1977) performed three interesting experiments with rats related to ulcer production. In one experiment, there were two groups of rats who received electric shocks. The A group learned to discriminate what was dangerous from what was safe (they learned when they would get shocks) and they had no, or very few stomach ulcers. The B group could not learn to discriminate; they had many stomach ulcers. The B group also had significantly higher corticoid levels than the A group. (B group had distress; A group had neustress?) In another experiment, the A group diminished the effectiveness of the shock by a coping response. In the B group, the rats were constantly frustrated and could not diminish the intensity of the shocks. The results showed that the B group had significantly higher corticoid levels and ulcers than the A group. In the third experiment, the A group was constantly under conflict as they had to take shocks to avoid getting more shocks. The B group was shocked regularly, but they had no conflicts. The results showed that the A group had significantly more stomach ulcers and higher steroid levels than the B group.

Cortisone acts on the blood vessels of the kidney, causing contraction and release of pressor* substances, such as renin. The latter causes a systemic rise in blood pressure, which, if continued, results in persistent hypertension.

Excess corticosteroids also act on the intestinal tract to inhibit the activity of vitamin D. This interferes with the absorption of calcium and can lead to bone resorption.

During the stress response, the anterior pituitary releases a third hormone called *thyrotrophin-stimulating hormone* (TSH) into the blood stream. This, in turn, stimulates the thyroid gland to release thyroid hormones that accelerate the body's metabolism. This response is beneficial for normal stress responses, such as those accompanying exercise. But it could become damaging from chronic stress responses and might lead to the development of hyperthyroidism.

Autonomic Nervous System Response

The stressor message to the hypothalamus also activates the autonomic nervous system, principally the sympathetic division. This causes the release of epinephrine (adrenaline) and norepinephrine (noradrenaline) from sympathetic nerve endings and epinephrine (principally) from the adrenal medulla. There is some evidence that ACTH also activates the release of epinephrine from the adrenal medulla. The action of epinephrine and norepinephrine (catecholamines) results in increases in blood pressure and blood glucose, dilation of the bronchioles, and irritation of the lining of the digestive tract. Animal experiments by Miller (1977) has shown that with brief episodes of fear there is a decrease of gastric HCl; with chronic fear,

*A pressor is a substance that raises blood pressure.

there is an increased secretion of gastric HCl. These effects are added to the similar ones produced by the corticoids. In addition, the catecholamines cause other reactions that are part of the fight-or-flight response described by Walter Cannon (1914). These reactions are (1) an increase in cardiac activity that can lead to irregular heart sounds (arrhythmias);* (2) increased heart rate (can lead to tachycardia);* (3) increased motor nerve excitability; (4) increased sweating of the palms and soles (measured as decreased skin resistance); (5) increased respiratory rate, minute ventilation, oxygen consumption, and carbon dioxide elimination (the chest expands and the throat relaxes to allow for the increased gaseous exchange); (6) dilation of the pupils (allows for increased visual perception); (7) decreased salivation, but of a more viscous type of "ropy" saliva (Box 1-9); (8) increased blood lactate (breakdown product of glucose); (9) increased blood cholesterol and free fatty acids (if repeated, could aggravate coronary arteries and lead to atherosclerosis); (10) increased uric acid (under certain chronic conditions could lead to gout); and (11) transfer of blood flow from the intestines and skin to the heart and skeletal muscles (important for muscular work).

Not everyone shows all of the reactions. Some people react primarily with increased breathing rate, others show principally an elevated blood pressure, still others have a more rapid heart rate, and some have increased palmar sweating. There is also evidence that under different types of stressors there are slightly different responses. The physical stressor of exercising shows different responses if the subjects experience different emotions while exercising (Box 1-10). There are also different responses when the stress is chronic.

Box 1-9: The Perils of Being Dry

The Arabian Bedouins formerly required conflicting witnesses to a crime to lick a hot iron. The witness whose tongue was burned was considered to be the liar. The ancient Chinese purportedly made an individual under interrogation

*More likely after repeated episodes of stress.

chew rice powder and then spit it out. If the expectorated powder came out dry, then the suspect was judged to be guilty. Years ago, in Great Britain, a suspect was given a "trial slice" of bread and cheese. If he could not swallow that combination, he was found guilty. In all of these cases, the guilty verdict was based on the common observation that when a person is under stress, his salivation diminishes until his mouth becomes dry (Smith, 1967).

Dentists observe a similar phenomenon with patients under stress. Unfortunately, the decrease in salivation is often accompanied by a conversion of the remaining saliva into a thick, ropy, mucilaginous type; the type that usually sticks to dentists' hands.

Box 1-10: Exercising While Emoting and Shocking While Petting

In a study discussed by Gary Schwartz (1977), subjects had somewhat different responses to exercise if subjectively they had feelings of anger, fear, happiness, jubilation, sadness, or if they meditated while exercising. This may account for the apparent better physiologic responses during eustress, as compared to distress.

Another example showing that moods can affect the stress response was reported by James Page (1971). It was observed that petting a dog while the animal is simultaneously being shocked decreases the severity of the expected cardiovascular responses. Apparently, the petting resulted in the dog becoming tranquil or happy, which in turn affected the physiological stress responses. The results also showed that the subjective responses were probably altered. That is, the petted-shocked dogs often showed no overt signs of being shocked.

Selye (1976) described the general adaptation syndrome (GAS). In the first stage, acute stress (or the alarm reaction), the previously described responses occur (H-AP-AC axis and autonomic nervous system response). In the second stage, resistance to stress, the body adapts to the chronic stressors, and there is a decreased corticoid level (and presumably also catecholamine level). In the third stage, exhaustion (fatigue), in which physiological reactions are no longer sufficient for adjusting to the stress, there is the highest level of corticoids (and probably catecholamines), and the body then is likely to succumb to serious disease and death.

Although the sympathetic nervous system is the predominant one activated during stress, there is also some parasympathetic action that generally dampens down the sympathetic response, e.g. lowers blood pressure and pulse rate. As mentioned previously, in certain individuals, parasympathetic activity predominates during the stress response (vagotonics). Reactions seen in these individuals include cold sweating, decreased blood pressure and heart rate, nausea, dizziness, and fainting. In certain instances, serious or even fatal reactions can occur.

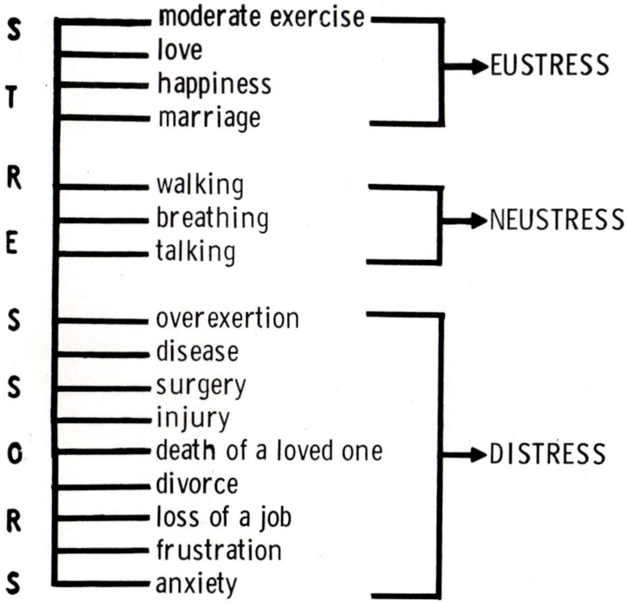

Figure 1-2. The interrelationship of some stressors and stress responses.

The interrelationship of some stressors and stress responses is shown in Figure 1-2. Figure 1-3 is a representation of the physiological changes during stress. Precursors of epinephrine and norepinephrine are found in the brain, and as mentioned previously, they may be involved with the activation of the stress reaction (along with the prostaglandins). The formation of epinephrine from tyrosine (an amino acid) is shown in Figure 1-4. It can be noted from the figure that ACTH and the corticoids are involved in the formation of epinephrine, showing that the two stress systems (the H-AP-AC and autonomic nervous systems) are interrelated.

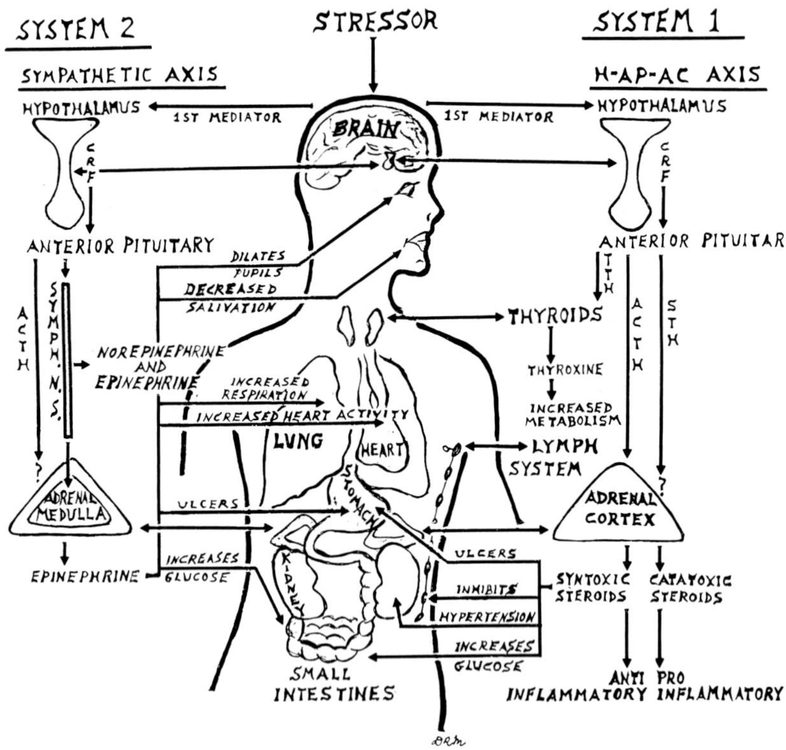

Figure 1-3. The stress response.

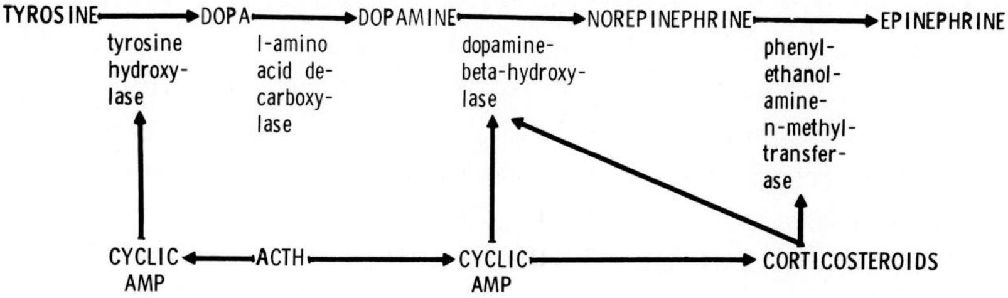

Figure 1-4. Pathways of epinephrine biosynthesis showing the interrelationship of the stress systems.

Psychological Responses and Objective Signs

When people are stressed, there are certain subjective responses and objective signs. All of these manifestations are not always seen, and they may occur randomly. Some responses are trembling, shaking, or fidgeting; feeling giddy, "high," confused, or even drunk; having heart palpitations (feeling as if the heart will leap out of the chest); having a "sinking" feeling in the stomach; and perspiring, blushing, and generally having feelings of anxiety. If one tries to talk, his speech may show hesitation, quivering, speed, or stammering.

In part, the manifestations of stress are related to whether neustress, eustress, or distress is generated. With distress, people may vomit or even urinate and defecate. The stress responses can also vary from a sympathetic to a parasympathetic response, e.g. from an elevated blood pressure and rapid pulse to a slow, feeble pulse, low blood pressure, and fainting.

Both the physiological and psychological responses of stress have recently been used in popular technology to evaluate when people are under stress (Box 1-11).

Summary

It appears that the type of stress response generated depends upon the strength and duration of the stressor and the makeup of the respondent. The more severe and repetitious the stressors are, the greater the chance for distress and eventual disease. The more fit the individual is in terms of physical condition, mental awareness, and ability to relax (in appropriate situations), the greater the chance for eustress and the promotion of good health.

One method that can be used to mitigate against the harmful effects of stressors is initiation of the relaxation response (*see* Chaps. 5 and 6). Other methods, such as avoidance of stressors, mental and physical preparation, and exercise, are discussed in Chapter 6.

Box 1-11: Detecting Lies and Moods

The polygraph (lie detector) is a well-known instrument used to evaluate certain physiological responses that change in a characteristic manner when an individual is under stress. The standard commercial polygraph records pulse rate, blood pressure, the rate and depth of breathing, and skin resistance. The rationale of the lie detector is based on the assumption that when a person lies his effort at deception is accompanied by emotional responses, such as anxiety, fear, and guilt. These psychological stressors induce typical reactions of the stress response, such as increased heart and breathing rate and decreased skin resistance. However, some individuals can fool the lie dector while they are being questioned by tensing or relaxing muscles or by concentrating on mental images. Also, some people show slight changes in physiological measures, even if they are severely stressed. In addition, the quality of polygraph operators varies greatly. Capable operators can easily detect objective signs of stress, such as fidgeting, stammering, hesitation, and blushing. Less capable practitioners may miss some of these stress-related clues. As a result, the lie detector test cannot be universally applied (Smith, 1967).

Recently, a popular version of the lie detector has surfaced. A Radio Shack flyer has offered a pocket lie detector kit for $11.95. The ad suggests that you can "Test your family, friends, party-goers! — Fingertip sensors reveal body changes due to nervousness" (Radio Shack, 1978).

Another recent innovation is the Hagoth®. This hand-held instrument is a miniature version of a *psychological stress evaluation* (PSE). The Hagoth supposedly can determine when a person is lying by measuring the amount of stress in his speech. This instrument is being promoted to business executives and sells for $1,500. With it, one can monitor friend and foe alike during routine telephone conversations. The person being monitored is completely unaware that anything unusual is taking place.

Israel has developed an instrument that is used to screen persons crossing the borders. The gadget measures an individual's chest cavity from a short distance. The concept is that variations from normal give an indication of changes in blood pressure and respiratory rate (Oster, 1978).

In the mid-1970s, stress was measured for a different purpose, using another technique. During those years, the mood ring became popular. The changing colors of the ring were supposed to indicate a person's physiological and subjective state. For example, when the ring turned black or dark blue, this was interpreted to mean that the person felt either sad, dejected, or depressed. In contradistinction, a yellow color was considered to mean that the individual concerned was calm, relaxed, and happy. Within the ring were cholesteric crystals, which changed colors with variations in skin temperature. The mood ring was based on the physiological blood flow changes that occur during stress and relaxation. With the stress response, there is peripheral vasoconstriction, a decreased skin temperature, and cold extremities. With the relaxation response, there is peripheral vasodilation, an increased skin temperature, and warm extremities. Outdoor temperatures could also affect the mood ring, and the enclosed crystals were quite fragile. These two factors probably accounted for the rapid demise of the mood rings.

RELAXATION

Introduction

As stated earlier, there have been well over 100,000 medical publications on stress. In comparison, little scientific writing has dealt with relaxation. Nevertheless, almost as much is known about the relaxation response as is known about the stress response. Before considering the relaxation response, a definition of *relaxation* is developed. Relaxation is also a term used in physics. It means the return of a system to equilibrium following displacement. In biology, the meaning is somewhat similar, especially when one considers *muscular relaxation,* the lengthening of a muscle or muscle fibers. It is the opposite of *muscular contraction,* the shortening of a muscle or muscle fibers. *Displacement* in physics terminology is comparable to *contraction* in biology; *return to equilibrium* in physics is *relaxation* in biology. Muscular relaxation also means the state of being lax or loose. It applies to skin as well as to muscles.

Mental relaxation means that the mind is at ease, at rest, or relieved from strain or effort. Mental and physical relaxation often occur simultaneously, but it is possible to be relaxed physically and still have an active mind. (This was found to be true in the physiological studies on relaxation techniques undertaken by the authors, Morse et al., 1977).

One can also exercise (for example, jog) and still be relaxed mentally. Mental and physical relaxation can occur separately or be combined as during periods of sleep, hypnosis, and meditation.

One can counteract the effects of distress in two ways: (1) by stimulating the parasympathetic nervous system, which causes reactions opposite to those produced by the sympathetic nervous system; and (2) by decreasing the activity of the sympathetic nervous system. Certain methods appear to achieve these responses, including rest, simple relaxation, sleep, quiet music, massage, and types of bathing. Drugs can also be used. However, a generally safe, effective, and reliable way to alter the autonomic responses is to initiate the relaxation response.

Relaxation Response

Over twenty years ago, Walter Hess (1957) first described the *trophotropic response.* He considered it to be "a protective mechanism against overstress . . . [which] are opposed to ergotropic reactions which are oriented toward increased oxidative metabolism and utilization of energy." The *ergotropic reactions* of Hess corresponds to the fight-or-flight sympathetic stress response of Cannon. The trophotropic response results from decreased sympathetic nervous system activity and increased parasympathetic activity, and it corresponds to the *relaxation response* of Benson (Box 1-12).

Box 1-12: The Relaxation Response

The responses that Hess observed in experiments with cats included decreased blood pressure and respiratory rate and constriction of the pupils. Benson recently investigated the human counterpart of this trophotropic response and concluded that it can be achieved by deep relaxation such as that achieved during Transcendental Meditation (TM). He called the reaction the relaxation response. Benson's investigations showed that this response could be achieved by various relaxation techniques in addition to TM, including simple-word meditation, Yoga and Zen meditation, relaxation-hypnosis, progressive relaxation, autogenic training, cotention, sentic cycles, and religious prayer (Benson, 1974).

Just as the stress response is brought on by stressors, the techniques that elicit the relaxation response can be called *relaxors.*

Relaxors

The definition of a relaxor is similar to that of a stressor. Relaxors are any physical, psychological, or social techniques that have the potentiality to induce certain physiological and psychological changes in a given individual at a particular time. Collectively, the changes are known as the relaxation response. It appears that the relaxation response is an important mechanism in enabling individuals to cope with the overabundance of stressors that accompany modern living. The type and duration of the relaxor, e.g. how long it is practiced per day, and the specific makeup of the individual (normal, neurotic, or psychotic) determine how he reacts to the relaxor. As with stress, responses can be neutral, favorable, or unfavorable. An example of a neutral response is the rested feeling following an average morning meditation; a favorable response is the euphoric feeling immediately after a "good" late-afternoon meditation; a negative response following meditation is the feeling of loss of control that can lead to a psychotic break* in susceptible individuals. The components and techniques of the various relaxors are discussed in Chapter 5.

Individual Makeup

Although the mediating and conditioning factors have been studied in relationship to stress, little investigation has been done on the relationship of the relaxation response to different types of individuals. As discussed previously, there are major personality differences between people, e.g. extroverts versus introverts and "uppers" versus "downers." People also vary in their autonomic nervous system responses to stress, e.g. sympatheticotonics, vagotonics, and normal responders. These individual variations could modify the type and extent of the relaxor used. Other factors that could affect the choice of relaxor are age, sex, diet, disease, drug intake, physical fitness, mental capacity, biorhythm, brain laterality, occupation, and family situation. One form of relaxor is simple-word meditation (Box 1-13; *see* Chap. 5).

Box 1-13: I Love That "Grik"

Recently, Patricia Carrington (1977) at Princeton and the authors' group at Temple University has shown that the effectiveness of certain words and sounds for meditation ap-

---

*Meditation or hypnosis can bring forth symptoms of severe mental disease in susceptible individuals.

pears to be related to personality. For example, most people do better with pleasant-sounding and emotionally positive words and sounds, such as *love* and *lohm*. Yet, a large minority of people tested (37% in our study) had a better response with unpleasant and negatively charged words and sounds, such as *hate* and *grik*. The responses also appeared to be correlated with personality types. Carrington found some evidence that people who are depressed have beneficial results from using the unpleasant-sounding "grik." The use of this sound may help those individuals get rid of their negative feelings.

It appears that the length of duration of the relaxor varies with different people. For example, some individuals receive maximum effectiveness from ten minutes of meditation, while others require at least twenty minutes. It also seems that when people are ill in bed, they derive benefit from longer periods of meditation. Paradoxically, when the same people are well, long periods of meditation can be upsetting. The time of day to use the technique and the number of relaxors used per day, e.g. one or two meditations, may be related to personality. There also can be a relationship between physique and metabolism and the type and duration of relaxor to be used.

Finally, it seems that relaxors should be avoided by certain individuals. For example, for people who fear loss of control or dislike being left alone, a relaxor such as self-hypnosis or meditation can bring forth extreme anxiety. There are various other outlets, some of which can be used for these people. These outlets include drug therapy, e.g. tranquilizers, psychologic and religious consultations, exercise, reading, traveling, hobbies, and so on. These are discussed in Chapters 5 and 6. The physiology and psychology of the relaxation response are considered next.

Changes Induced by the Relaxation Response

Physiological Responses

As with stress, the relaxation response is initiated in the

hypothalamus (also verified by electrical stimulation experimentally; Benson, 1974). Some unknown signal causes activation of the parasympathetic nervous system (responses are generally opposite to those of the sympathetic nervous system) and deactivation of the sympathetic nervous system. It is not known if the H-AP-AC axis is involved. However, considering the relationship of the autonomic nervous system and the H-AP-AC axis with stress, it appears that activation of the relaxation response cuts down the release of syntoxic steroids and thyroid hormones (Box 1-14).

Box 1-14: The "Guts" of Meditation

Physiological studies by Wallace (1970), Benson (1974) and the authors' group at Temple University (1977), have shown the following reactions to be indicative of the relaxation response: (1) decreased oxygen consumption, carbon dioxide elimination, respiratory rate, minute ventilation, sweating of the palms and soles (increased skin resistance), blood cholesterol, skeletal muscle activity, and blood flow to the skeletal muscles (as contrasted to the flow during stress; (2) increased alpha and (occasionally) theta brain wave patterns; and (3) constriction of the pupils (visual acuity is not needed). Although blood pressure does not change significantly, if there is continued practice of the relaxation response over a period of months, then there are significant decreases in blood pressure.

Figure 1-5 is a diagrammatic representation of the physiological changes during the relaxation response.

Psychological Responses and Objective Signs

Subjective feelings described for the relaxation response vary with individuals, the time of day the technique is practiced, and the type of technique practiced. However, there are certain feelings that are often expressed. These include floating, warmth, tingling, numbness, out-of-body sensation, dissocia-

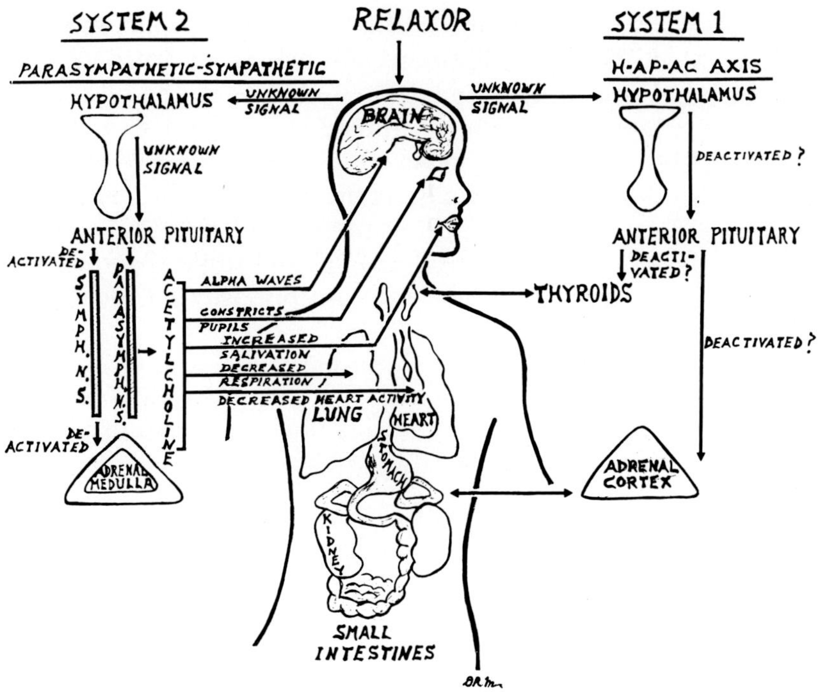

Figure 1-5. The relaxation response.

tion, euphoria, and various mental images. The subjects often state that they cannot hear their heartbeats and are unaware of their breathing. They generally verbalize feelings of peace and tranquility. The people look relaxed; their arms and legs hang loosely and their facial and scalp muscles are unwrinkled. If their eyes are open (as can occur during hypnosis), they may look "spaced out."

Summary

Relaxation is an important and effective means of counteracting the results of continual exposure to stressors that occur with current life-styles. Although relaxation can be achieved by simply relaxing, daydreaming, napping, or sleeping, a far more effective and predictable method is to elicit the relaxation response. Meditation and hypnosis are two easily learned techniques that bring forth this response. Although the relaxation response is beneficial for most individuals, there are variations that must be considered in relation to personality and physical types. For certain individuals, detrimental results can occur from the use of the relaxation response, and alternative methods should be used. The physiological and subjective manifestations of the relaxation response are opposite to those seen with stress.

In the remaining chapters, consideration is given to the dental role of stress, relaxation, and other coping methods. Chapter 2 begins with a discussion of the dental patient's stress.

REFERENCES

Adler, A.: *Study of Organ Inferiority and its Psychical Compensation.* Washington, D. C., Nervous and Mental Disease Publishing Co., 1917.

Antelman, S. M. and Caggiula, A. R.: Norepinephrine-dopamine interactions and behavior. *Science, 195:*646, 1977.

Beary, J. F. and Benson, H.: A simple psychophysiologic technique which elicits the hypometabolic changes of the relaxation response. *Psychosom Med, 36:*115, 1974.

Beecher, H. K.: Relationship of significance of wound to the pain experienced. *JAMA, 161:*1609, 1956.

Becker, B. J.: A holistic approach to anxiety and stress. *Am J Psychoanal, 36:*139, 1976.

Benson, H.: Your innate asset for combatting stress. *Harvard Bus Rev, 52(4):*49, 1974.

____: *The Relaxation Response: An Innate Capacity for Dealing With Stress.* Read before the Symposium on Stress and Behavioral Medicine. New York, Dec. 3-4, 1977a.

____: Systemic hypertension and the relaxation response. *N Engl J Med, 296:*1152, 1977b.

Benson, H., Beary, J. F., and Carol, M. P.: The relaxation response. *Psychiatry, 37:*37, 1974.

Benson, H., Kotch, J. B., and Crassweller, R. D.: The relaxation response: A bridge between psychiatry and medicine. *Med Clin North Am, 61:*929, 1977.

Borland, L. R.: Odontophobia — Inordinate fear of dental treatment. *Dent*

*Clin North Am, 6:*683, 1962.

Brown, W. A. and Heninger, G.: Stress-induced growth hormone release: Psychologic and physiologic correlates. *Psychosom Med, 38:*145, 1976.

Cannon, W. B.: The emergency function of the adrenal medulla in pain and the major emotions. *Am J Physiol, 33:*356, 1914.

Carrington, P.: *New Directions in Meditation Research.* Read before the Symposium on Meditation Related Therapies. St. Louis, Oct. 28-29, 1977.

Christie, M. J. and Venables, P. H.: Change in palmar skin potential level during relaxation after stress. *J Psychosom Res, 18:*301, 1974.

Crasilneck, H. B. and Hall, J. A.: Physiological changes associated with hypnosis: A review of the literature since 1948. *Int J Clin Exp Hypn, 7:*9, 1959.

Editorial: Just relax! — Transcendental Meditation reduces cholesterol level. *Jewish Press, 27(40):*53, Oct. 7, 1977.

Eliot, R. S.: Stress and cardiovascular disease. *Eur J Cardiol, 5(2):*97, 1977.

Erikson, E. H.: *Childhood and Society.* New York, Norton, 1950.

Glass, D. C.: Stress, behavior patterns and coronary disease. *Am Sci, 65:*177, 1977.

Hanukoglu, I.: Prostaglandins as first mediators of stress? *Lancet, 1:*193, 1977.

Hedge, G. A.: Roles for prostaglandins in the regulation of anterior pituitary secretion. *Life Sci, 20:*17, 1977.

Hess, W. R.: *The Functional Organization of the Diencephalon.* New York, Grune, 1957.

Hilgard, E. R. and Hilgard, J. A.: *Hypnosis in the Relief of Pain.* Los Altos, Calif., William Kaufman, 1975, pp. 32-33.

Hodges, R. E.: The effect of stress on ascorbic acid metabolism in man. *Nutr Today, 5(1):*11, 1970.

Hurst, M. W., Jenkins, C. D., and Rose, R. M.: The relationship of psychological stress to onset of medical illness. In Creger, W. P., Coggins, C. H., and Hancock, E. W. (Eds.): *Ann Rev Med, 27:*301, 1976.

Jung, C. G.: *Psychological Types.* New York, Harcourt Brace and World, 1923.

Kagan, A.: A stressless definition of "stress" and some speculations on its relationship to cardiovascular disease. *Acta Cardiol (Brux), 30:*331, 1975.

Kehlet, H., Brandt, M., Enquist, A., and Medsen, S. N.: Prostaglandins as mediators of stress reaction. *N Engl J Med, 297(12):*672, 1977.

Kopin, I. J.: Catecholamines, adrenal hormones, and stress. *Hosp Pract, 11:*49, Mar., 1976.

Krueger, A. P. and Reed, E. J.: Biological impact of small air ions. *Science, 193:*1209, 1976.

Lazarus, R. S.: *Coping With Stress: Effects on Somatic Illness, Morale, and Social Functioning.* Read before the Symposium on Stress and Behavioral Medicine. New York, Dec. 3-4, 1977.

Leff, D. N.: Doctors debate brain: Controversy flares over use of endorphins on patients. *Med World News, 19:*86-96, Jan. 9, 1978.

Miller, N. E.: Liberalization of basic S-R concept: Extensions to conflict behavior, motivation, and social learning. In Koch, S. (Ed.): *Psychology: A study of a science.* Vol. 2. New York, McGraw, 1959, pp. 196-292.

Miller, N. E.: *Learning Effects on Somatic Manifestations of Stress.* Read before the Symposium on Stress and Behavioral Medicine. New York, Dec. 3-4, 1977.

Miller, N. E. and Dworkin, B. R.: Effects of learning on visceral functions — Biofeedback. *N Engl J Med, 296:*1274, 1977.

Monjan, A. A. and Collector, M. I.: Stress-induced modulation of the immune response. *Science, 196:*307, 1977.

Morse, D. R.: *Clinical Endodontology: A Comprehensive Guide to Diagnosis, Treatment and Prevention.* Springfield, Ill., Thomas, 1974, p. 6.

Morse, D. R., Martin, J. S., Furst, M. L., and Dubin, L. L.: A physiological and subjective evaluation of meditation, hypnosis and relaxation. *Psychosom Med, 39:*304, 1977.

Noel, G. R., Dimond, R. C., Earll, J. M., and Frantz, A. G.: Prolactin, thyrotropin, and growth hormone release during stress associated with parachute jumping. *Aviat Space Environ Med, 47:*543, 1976.

Orme-Johnson, D. W.: Autonomic stability and transcendental meditation. *Psychosom Med, 35:*341, 1973.

Oster, P.: Technology, Big Brother are invading your privacy. *Philadelphia Evening Bulletin,* sec. 1b, p. 10, Jan. 10, 1978.

Page, J. D.: *Psychopathology: The Science of Understanding Deviance.* Chicago, Aldine-Atherton, 1971.

Perchellet, J. P., Shanker, G., and Sharma, R. K.: Regulatory role of guanosine 3′, 5′-monophosphate in adrenocorticotropin hormone-induced steroidogenesis. *Science, 199:*311, 1978.

Petrich, J. and Holmes, T. H.: Life change and onset of illness. *Med Clin North Am, 61:*825, 1977.

Piaget, J.: *The Construction of Reality in the Child.* New York, Basic, 1954.

Rabkin, J. G. and Struening, E. L.: Life events, stress and illness. *Science, 194:*1013, 1976.

Radio Shack Catalog No. 289: Pocket lie detector kit, 143, 1978.

Rahe, R. H.: *Life Stress Events and Illness.* Read before the Symposium on Stress and Behavioral Medicine. New York, Dec. 3-4, 1977.

Rahe, R. H., Ryman, D. H., and Biersner, R. J.: Serum uric acid, cholesterol, and psychological moods throughout stressful naval training. *Aviat Space Environ Med, 47:*883, 1976.

Rees, W. L.: Stress, distress and disease. *Br J Psychiatry, 128:*3, 1976.

Rotter, J. B.: Generalized expectancies for internal versus external control of reinforcement. *Psychol Monogr, 80(609),* 1966.

Samples, R. E.: Learning with the whole brain. *Hum Behav, 4(2):*16, 1975.

Schlesinger, J., Barzilay, J., Stryjer, D., and Almog, C. H.: Life threatening "vagal reaction" to emotional stimuli. *Isr J Med Sci, 13:*59, 1977.

Schwartz, G. E.: *The Brain as a Health Care System: A Psychobiological Foundation for Stress and Behavioral Medicine.* Read before the Symposium on Stress and Behavioral Medicine. New York, Dec. 3-4, 1977.

Seifter, E.: Of stress, vitamin A, and tumors. *Science, 193:*74, 1976.

Seltzer, S.: *Endodontology: Biologic Considerations in Endodontic Procedures.* New York, McGraw, 1971, p. 408.

Selye, H.: *Stress Without Distress.* Philadelphia, Lippincott, 1974.

——: Further thoughts on "stress without distress." *Med Times, 104(11):*124, 1976a.

——: *The Stress of Life,* 2nd ed. New York, McGraw, 1976b.

——: Stress without distress: Evolution of the functional concept. Read before the Symposium on Stress and Behavioral Medicine. New York, Dec. 3-4, 1977.

Sheehy, G.: *Passages: Predictable Crises of Adult Life.* New York, Dutton, 1976.

Sheldon, W. H.: *Atlas of Men: A Guide for Somatotyping the Adult Male at All Ages.* New York, Harper, 1954.

Smith, B. M.: The polygraph. *Sci Am, 216 (1):*25, 1967.

Solomon, R. L. and Brush, E. S.: Experimentally derived conceptions of anxiety and aversion. In Jones, M. R. (Ed.): *Nebraska Symposium on Motivation.* Lincoln, U of Neb Pr, 1956.

Stone, R. A. and DeLeo, J.: Psychotherapeutic control of hypertension. *N Engl J Med, 294:*80, 1976.

Stoyva, J.: *Cultivated Low Arousal Through Biofeedback: A Learned Anti-stress Response?* Read before the Symposium on Stress and Behavioral Medicine. New York, Dec. 3-4, 1977.

Stumpf, W. E. and Sar, M.: The heart: A target organ for estradiol. *Science, 196:*319, 1977.

Syvalahti, E., Lammintausta, R., and Pekkarinen, A.: Effect of psychic stress of examination on serum growth hormone, serum insulin, and plasma renin activity. *Acta Pharmacol Toxicol (Kbh), 38:*344, 1976.

Wallace, R. K.: Physiological effects of transcendental meditation. *Science, 167:*1751, 1970.

Walrath, L. C., and Hamilton, D. W.: Autonomic correlates of meditation and hypnosis. *Am J Clin Hypn, 17:*190, 1975.

Young, L. D., Langford, H. G., and Blanchard, E. G.: Effect of operant conditioning of heart rate on plasma renin activity. *Psychosom Med, 38:*278, 1976.

CHAPTER 2

THE PATIENT'S STRESS

The relationship of patient stress to fear and the dental office situation is covered. The differences between fear, anxiety, panic, and phobia are considered. The three causes of dental fear, dental experiences, the psychosexual significance of the mouth, and the self-image, are examined in detail. A questionnaire to assess patient's dental fears is presented. The relationship of stress and oral diseases is evaluated.

STRESS AND DENTAL TREATMENT

Introduction

IT'S 5:15 PM and your mind wanders to the events of the day. At 8:45 AM, Mildred enters: "Dr. Pierce, Mrs. Jaffe cancelled her nine o'clock appointment; something about her sick daughter; and that was her third straight missed appointment." At 9:30 Mrs. Cordova brings in her screaming, kicking, lovable child, Jeffrey. It takes the two assistants, the receptionist, Mrs. Cordova, and yourself just to put a mirror in his mouth. And you hear her exclaim as she carries him out, "You'll see, you're gonna wind up with plates, just like your father, you stupid brat!" Ten o'clock isn't too bad. After all, Mr. Greene only spits out eight times while you put in that occlusal amalgam. In addition, you required just three towels to dispose of his sweat. But 10:30, that's a different story. "Thank God, it was only a small cut. Oh, why couldn't Jackie keep his head still!" Still, it could've been worse; you did manage to stop the bleeding. The consultation with Mr. Margolis at 11:00 would have been fine if you could have gotten a word in edgewise. "I wonder if he'll accept the treatment plan!" Well, at least you get a break at 11:30. "I can't believe it; the guy called me at 3:00 in the morning saying he was in excruciating pain; so we squeeze him in, and he doesn't show up; and not even a call. The toothache must have stopped. When will they ever learn?!" Lunch is great; a new variety, banana yogurt. Then the one o'clock patient, Miss Peters, comes in. She looks okay, "Just a little pale!" But as soon as she sees the needle, out she goes. It isn't all bad. When she comes to, she apologizes and makes another appointment. Freddie at 1:30 accidentally(?) bites your finger. "Heck, it hardly hurts now!" Then at 2:00, you have that robot, Frank Irving. "Gee, he didn't say two words for the whole hour appointment." Three o'clock is a fun festival. But fat Frieda never stops laughing (aside from a few tears) and you do get to finish *two* whole surfaces. Tanya at 3:30 is ideal. So what if she needed nitrous, Valium®, a little hypnosis, and two and one-half Carpules® of Xylocaine®. Mrs. Adams is very cooperative, on time at four, and really no problem, but she still owes you $375. It's good that you saved the 4:30 slot for a "problem" patient. So you can't really complain about Mr. Vetch. Anyway his punch is wide. But it's not so bad, you've had worse days than this one . . . or have you?

Although these recollections of a typical dentist's day may be exaggerated, all of the patient responses described are related to patient stress. The principal cause of patient stress is fear. In the remainder of this section is an exploration of the types and causes of patients' stress. Although fear and anxiety are the foremost factors, there are other considerations related to the dental office that cause patient distress.

Fear is derived from the old English term *faer,* meaning sudden calamity or danger. It is a normal response that entails feelings of alarm or disquiet caused by the realistic expectation of danger, pain, or disaster, e.g. being frightened at the sight of a needle.

Anxiety is derived from the Greek word meaning "to press tight" or "to strangle." It is a response that engenders feelings indistinguishable from fear, but it is brought on by a source of danger that is vague. The anxious person has intense fear or dread, but there is no realistic object or situation that engenders the fear. There are two types of anxiety. The first is *generalized trait anxiety,* in which the individual experiences anxiety as a personality characteristic or as a stable aspect of his life-style. He is anxious about every new situation. The second type of anxiety is *transitional situational anxiety,* in which a generally nonanxious person could temporarily feel anxious because of a specific occasion or potentially stressful occurrence. Dental anxiety, which is the fear of having dental treatment performed without really knowing why, could be manifested in either individual. However, it is often brought on by hearing "tales of woe" or "horror stories" from other people.

Panic is derived from the word for the Greek god Pan, who was the originator of sudden and unexplainable terror. Panic means a sudden surge of intense terror; it can occur with any condition that causes severe anxiety. (Most people have seen panic-stricken patients in the reception rooms of dentists.)

Phobia is derived from the word for the Greek god Phobos, who provoked panic and flight in his enemies. A phobia is a persistent, abnormal, or illogical fear. It is out of proportion to the object or situation feared and results in avoidance of the feared situation or object. There are many people who never go to the dentist because of dental phobias. An example is the person who avoids the dentist because of the traumatic childhood memory of a painful extraction.

Dental Fear*

Your tongue begins a probing action; suddenly it feels something sharp and jagged. It then descends into a great ravine, and you scream in pain and fear. The uncovered chasm is a "cavity," and it is difficult to separate the real from the anticipated hurt. You also know the discovery means a trip to the dentist or, alternatively, the agonies of a toothache. And you are in a quandary, because you do not know which is the lesser evil. If you are like the average American, there's a fifty-fifty chance that you will sit home and suffer for a time rather than make that fateful call to the dentist. And why is this the case?

*The term *fear* is used throughout the book with the understanding that in specific cases, either fear, anxiety, phobia, or panic is the more appropriate term.

There is an overriding fear of dental treatment. Fear of dentistry is among the most common of all fears in our present society.

In William Goldman's (1974) novel, *Marathon Man,* the hero Babe described dental fear succinctly: "It was all very primitive. It went beyond pain. The dentist meant fear." In fact, dental fear is so widespread that one of the reasons the movie version of this novel probably did not do better financially was that prospective moviegoers stayed away in droves because of the descriptive stories they heard from others about the dental "torture" scenes. Dental fear is related to three factors: The first is dental experiences; the second is the psychosexual significance of the oral cavity; and the third is the location of the self.

Dental Experiences

People often get a bad image of dentistry from talking with others. This generally occurs in the family situation. The parents' unpleasant oral experiences are related to the child, or the child might be present while his brother or sister has had a negative dental experience. Other reasons for dental fears or phobias are based on tales of horror told by friends, stories read, or movies seen. The media is a great purveyor of the terror of dental treatment.* Fear can also be based on the individual's own previous unfavorable dental or medical experiences, usually those that occurred in childhood (Box 2-1).

Box 2-1: Negative Experiences and Fear

Bernstein and Kleinknecht asked 225 college students to write an essay about their childhood experiences with dentistry and how they felt about dentists. Fifty-eight percent of the responses were negative, and the negative responses were higher with those who as adults had a great fear of dentistry. In another study, the same investigators observed 128 dental patients. They asked them to rate their dental fears on a scale from 1 (no fear) to 5 (high fear). The results showed that

*A good example of this is shown in the January, 1978, issue of *Psychology Today,* in which the dental chair is represented as an electric chair.

people who rated themselves as 5's were six times as liable to break or cancel appointments. It was also observed that patients over age forty (1) reported the least anxiety, (2) expected and had the least amount of pain, and (3) were least aroused physiologically at the end of the treatments. Their dentists rated these same patients as having the least pain (Hassett, 1978).

One dentally related fear is that of being gagged. People have seen movies in which individuals are gagged, and some may have been unfortunate enough to have had this occur to themselves. Gagging is a means of silencing or asphyxiating a person, and fear of this may be transferred to the dental office. Previously, in some dental offices (and possibly in some present-day offices) there was a practice to put a towel or a hand over the face of a screaming child. This was done in order to startle and immobilize the child enough so that some form of dental treatment could be performed. A second reason was to prevent the parent from hearing the screaming child and possibly run into the treatment room. Conceivably, some adult fears of suffocation could have been related to such incidents. Other adults had unpleasant childhood memories of masks over their faces for general anesthesia, which could also be transferred to dental fears of gagging, swallowing the tongue, or suffocation.

Other earlier unfavorable medical and dental childhood experiences that can be translated into adult fears are (1) being traumatized by the doctor or nurses "in white" (fear of the man in white) and (2) having a painful injection in the buttocks, arm, mouth or elsewhere in the body (fear of the needle).

Some patients have childhood memories of being scolded by the dentist because of dental neglect or not following instructions. This could deter them from seeking dental care as an adult because of the fear of a scolding repetition or because of guilt feelings for waiting so long.

Even if the patient had no previous fears of dental treatment, a rebuke by the dentist about his decrepit oral condition could initiate a negative self-image. The poor self-image could then be translated into fear of future dental treatment.

Another reason for dental fear is the early memory and history of a toothache. An adult may have conscious or subconscious recollections of teething. Pain is often associated with the eruption of teeth. The prospective adult patient might imagine that dental manipulation could cause pain of the same sort and, therefore, must be avoided. In this connection, Mark Twain's comment is apropos: "Adam and Eve had many advantages, but the principal one was that they escaped teething."

Although tooth eruption can cause a toothache, a cariously exposed pulp generally causes much more severe pain. A devastating toothache is never forgotten, although it may be deeply buried in the mind. Studies have shown that patients perceive oral pain as being more severe than pain from any other area of the body (Borland, 1962). This may be related to the proximity of the trigeminal nerve to the thalamus (pain reception center) and cerebral cortex (pain interpretation center). It is more likely, however, that the principal reason for dental pain being severe is the psychological importance of the oral cavity. Thus, an individual who once had a severe toothache might be reluctant to visit a dentist because of the fear that dental work would give rise to a similar toothache (Box 2-2).

Box 2-2: The Transcendental Toothache

The nineteenth century English poet Thomas Hood might have agreed that a toothache could disincline one from a dental visit when he wrote,

Of all our pains, since man was curst,
I mean of body, not the mental,
To name the worst, among the worst,
The dental sure is transcendental . . .

A traumatic dental experience may also give rise to dental fear. Dental injuries are quite prevalent, especially with the front teeth. They can occur as the result of contact sports (particularly, boxing and football) and sports accidents (especially hockey). Furthermore, front teeth are often broken, displaced, or avulsed (knocked out) by parents inflicting punishment on their children (the battered child syndrome).

Automobile and bathtub accidents often involve the teeth. An individual who has been in a serious accident where there was pain, bleeding, and swelling located in the mouth or face might be somewhat hesitant about going to a dentist. The hesitancy would be intensified, especially if the accident victim believed that the dental procedures themselves would be traumatic.

The fear of receiving trauma to the mouth is a deep-seated fear. It is related to the psychological significance of the mouth. If an individual wants to threaten someone else on a highly personal level, he threatens him orally. Examples are "I'll hit you in the mouth," "I'm gonna knock out all your teeth," or "I'm gonna knock your teeth down your throat." When one is hit in the jaw, bleeding occurs frequently. The oral cavity has one of the richest blood supplies of any area in the body, and oral bleeding can occur readily and be profuse. There are people who have a great fear of blood, particularly in their mouths. This might be related to incidents they have seen, such as oral bleeding during fights or bleeding as a result of internal injuries. It is possible that fear of bleeding could deter the patient from having regular dental care. Patients report having thoughts such as, "Will I stop bleeding when the tooth is pulled?" and "Will my gums bleed a lot when my teeth are cleaned?"

Psychosexual Significance of the Oral Cavity

On a sub- or semiconscious level (Box 2-3), the significance of the mouth is of great importance with dental fear.

Box 2-3: The Many-Faceted Mind

When terms such as *mind, subconscious, unconscious, semiconscious, superconscious,* and *cosmic consciousness* are used, they are not meant either in a literal or Freudian sense. Most of the time, the words are used because of current popularity. The basic notion communicated is that mental functioning occurs on other than the strictly conscious level.

The oral cavity is intimately concerned with almost all aspects of life from the time of birth to the time of death. Between the first breath of life and last dying gasp, a multitude of pleasurable activities is associated with the mouth. After the initial inhalation, a scream invariably follows. Screaming is considered to be an aggressive primal discharge of stress that instantly creates a bond with the protecting, sustaining parents of the extrauterine environment.

The next important activity of the infant, connecting with the external environment, is the (gratifying) sucking of a nipple. Sucking becomes a pleasurable, lifelong activity. Of course, the mother's nipple is used initially for gaining sustenance rather than for gratification. It is often followed by an artificial nipple and a pacifier. A child may substitute a lollipop or one of his fingers; an adult sucks on candy and fruit, and, during sexual play, on various body parts. Psychologically, thumb-sucking is considered to be the earliest autoerotic (oral) activity. The child uses his thumb as a stress-release mechanism, and other objects, e.g. cigars and pipes, are substituted in adult life. At times of stressful situations, some adults even revert (regress) to thumb-sucking.

Generally, biting is the next oral activity that follows. It is associated with the eruption of the primary dentition. Biting serves several purposes, including eating, pleasure, and stress release, and the teeth even serve as a weapon. With tooth eruption, the infant may inadvertently bite what he loves — the mother's breast — and by biting learns how to reject what he does not want. If carried into adulthood, a lover's ambivalent behavior may then be understood. Stress release may be obtained through nail-biting. Some psychiatrists consider this habit to be related both to oral sensual gratification and masochism. The latter aspect may resemble the destruction of part of one's self (the nails).

With tooth eruption comes the ability to eat solid foods. Undoubtedly, we eat to live, but too many people live to eat. Health authorities are agreed that a major health problem of people in the United States is obesity brought about by overeating.* As George Bernard Shaw said, "There is no love sincerer than the love of food." Eating, for many, is certainly one of life's true pleasures. The joys of eating are related to the taste, smell, and sensuous feel of the food. The oral cavity is one of the most highly innervated areas of the body. Oral taste, i.e. sweet, sour, salt, and bitter, and touch sensations are often transformed into pure pleasure. Consider the licking and tasting that goes on during eating, drinking, smoking, sucking, and sexual encounters. For many people, eating is also a means of relieving stress.

Although the child uses his teeth for biting and chewing while eating, chewing soon generates other pleasures. Chewing gum begins early in childhood and often continues throughout life. Chewing is pleasurable and is a method of stress release. Some adults substitute chewing tobacco for chewing gum.

Soon after a child learns the pleasures of eating, he is introduced to the joys of drinking. From chocolate milk to cola, from downing Scotch to the sipping of wine, the enjoyment found in drinking is well known. It is also known that people drink stimulants and alcoholic beverages not only for pleasure, but also for stress release.

The anticipation of something enjoyable, whether food, liquor, sex, or "sweet" revenge, sets in motion another pleasurable oral action — drooling. All people can recall when their mouths "watered" in anticipation. Even "spitting out" can have some pleasurable aspects, as with those who chew tobacco.

After eating or drinking, some of us belch with embarrassment. Although others may frown at this behavior, belching is usually a gratifying sensation and, in Oriental societies, it is considered a mark of good manners.

Aside from food and drink, the child soon learns either by watching his parents or by experimentation that exciting drugs may be taken by mouth. It is quickly found that many enjoyable sensations begin with the oral intake of tranquilizers, barbiturates, amphetamines, and hallucinogenic drugs.

---

*In a nationwide poll conducted by Alfred Politz Research, Inc., it was shown that "a total of 58% of all adults in America suffer from obesity in some degree" (Kordell, 1971).

When a child first begins to talk, it often is a trying experience. Soon, as he becomes competent, talking becomes enjoyable (unless he is shy or has a speech impediment). Many adults love to hear themselves talk and sing. Some people talk incessantly when under stress and sometimes they may be able to talk their way out of the stressful situation.

Whistling is another oral action that can be both enjoyable and a means of stress release, e.g. "whistling in the dark." Blowing is somewhat similar except teeth are not required, noise is not usually emitted, and more forceful lung action is necessary. Blowing ranges from simple enjoyment and stress release, e.g. blowing smoke rings and bubbles to sexual pleasures.

Another mouth action that is satisfying for many is smoking. Unfortunately, this is an activity that often begins in the teenage years. Whether people smoke cigarettes, cigars, pipes, or marijuana, enjoyment is one of the principal reasons for the habit. The sensual feel of the cigar or pipe on the lips and oral mucous membranes adds to the gratifying aspect of smoking. Undoubtedly, the smoking also provides stress release.

Kissing as a sign of affection begins early in a child's development. Early kisses are mere pecks, but later kissing during amorous exchanges involves the lips, tongue, cheeks, facial muscles, teeth, and saliva. Kissing is certainly one of the more pleasurable oral actions, especially when it is engaged in by emotionally involved couples.

Through mouth actions, pleasure can be expressed and communicated. Examples are smiling, laughing, and rolling of the tongue, e.g. as a sexual invitation. Associated with the sensuous importance attached to the mouth is the concern of men and women for esthetics. The beautiful smile of a Miss America, for example, may show meticulously placed lipstick and white, perfectly formed teeth.

When one considers the multitudinous nonfood objects that people put into their mouths, e.g. toys, thumbs, fingers, cigars, cigarettes, pipes, pencils, pens, toothpicks, swords, and sexual organs, it may be that from birth there is an almost innate desire to have something in the mouth.

According to psychoanalytic theory, the first phase in development is the *oral stage* (Cameron, 1963; and Hall, 1954). This begins in infancy when the head and mouth is physically much larger in proportion to the rest of the body than it is in the adult. In this period, the mouth is psychologically extremely important, since it is the introductory zone for the child's sense of reality; the child meets the world through the mouth. Freudians consider the mouth to be developmentally the first of three principal erogenous zones on the body (the other two are the anus and the genital organs).

The principal sources of oral pleasure are tactile, resulting from placing objects into the mouth, and biting. Within the psychoanalytic framework, tactile stimulation of the lips, tongue, cheeks, and palate by objects produces sexual pleasure. Biting, on the other hand, yields oral aggressive pleasures. Tactile pleasures tend to come first in development, because biting must await eruption of teeth. Infants elect to retain pleasurable objects, e.g. the mother's breast, and get rid of distasteful objects, e.g. bitter medicine. Therefore, they spit out that which they wish to reject. By learning from experience what is unsatisfactory, they ward off the bad taste or pain by keeping their mouths closed.

Freudians consider that infants function orally in five principal ways: (1) taking something in; (2) holding on to it; (3) biting it; (4) spitting it out; and (5) shutting the mouth against it. Each of these ways can be a prototype of a personality trait in an adult.

Taking something in is usually pleasurable. The individual who enjoys this mode may later in life revel in "taking in" or have "a hunger and thirst for" knowledge. The child who always "holds on" may become a determined, unyielding, or miserly individual (analogous to *retention* in the later anal stage). The infant who enjoys biting may become a destructive person. This oral aggression may evolve into "biting sarcasm," sadism, or masochism (self-punishment; lip, cheek, or tongue biting). The baby who spits out regularly can be the prototype of the rejecting and contemptuous adult. The child who keeps a closed mouth may develop into an individual with a closed mind, a person who keeps to himself.

Whether or not these infantile oral modes develop into adult personality traits depends upon the degree of anxiety and frustration that the infant experienced. For instance, a child may develop an adult tendency to hold tightly to everything if he was weaned off the nipple too soon.

It is also conceivable that people who always must have something in their mouths may be arrested at the oral stage of development. Again, according to the psychoanalytic model, the human mouth is a symbolic organ. The teeth symbolize potency and strength. The shape of the mouth is cavelike and symbolizes the vagina. There is more than a passing similarity between the mouth and the vagina. Both openings are protected by lips, both are relatively warm and moist, both are lined with pink mucous membranes, and the microbial flora is similar in both areas.

The close approximation of the mouth to the vagina, both physically and symbolically, gives a clue as to why some women patients resist invasion of a region in which so much pleasure is involved. There are women patients who subconsciously equate dental treatment with being raped. This is especially true if the treatment is abrupt and painful. Conversely, overzealous, kind handling of some women patients by male dentists may be perceived by the women as sexual advances. This is again related to the importance of the mouth in amorous exchanges and to its symbolism with the vagina.

There is some suggested Freudian symbolism between a tooth and the penis. Some men may subconsciously fear dental treatments because of the fear of the loss of teeth: This is equated with fear of castration.

Even for the average person, without considering abstruse Freudian interpretations, it is evident from the previous discussion of oral actions that the mouth is an important pleasure zone. People do not like to have their pleasures interfered with; hence, this is an important aspect of the fear of dental treatment.

The Self

Not only is the oral cavity important for pleasure reasons, it is also important because of its anatomical position. As mentioned previously, pain is felt more severely orally, and people dislike oral injections more intensely than anywhere else in the body. One reason stated before was the proximity of the trigeminal nerve to the central pain areas. A second and more important reason is the psychosexual significance of the oral cavity. The mouth is a highly personal area of gratification and as such should not be tampered with. But this is not the complete answer.

As part of a study, a question was posed to a group of subjects. They were asked, "Where in your body is the 'self'?" and "Where is your 'center'?" Most subjects answered, "My 'self' is located in the head area" (Borland, 1962). This response is reflected in how people react. Fear of intraoral injections was discussed before. The same is true for operations. The most stress-inducing operations are those in the face, mouth, or brain. It also related to appearance. Mothers become perturbed if a newborn child has a birth defect that is located in the head region and as a result is visible outside of clothing coverings. Problems that would be tolerated in the rest of the body cause distress if they are found in the head area. For example, cleft lip and severe malocclusion are two oral defects that cause parental and child consternation. The reason for the oral importance is because the mouth is considered to be close to the center of the self, and as such it must be kept inviolate.

There is an anatomical reason for the importance of the oral cavity. In the cerebral cortex, there is a large area representing sensory and motor innervation of the oral cavity. It is much larger than would be the case if representation was solely related to the size of the mouth in proportion to the rest of the body. A diagrammatic presentation of the relative size of mouth and cortex is found in Figure 2-1.

Expression of Fears

Knowing that dental fears are related to dental experiences, the psychosexual significance of the mouth and the location of the self, how these fears are expressed is now examined. Fear of the unknown (not knowing what will happen), is what keeps

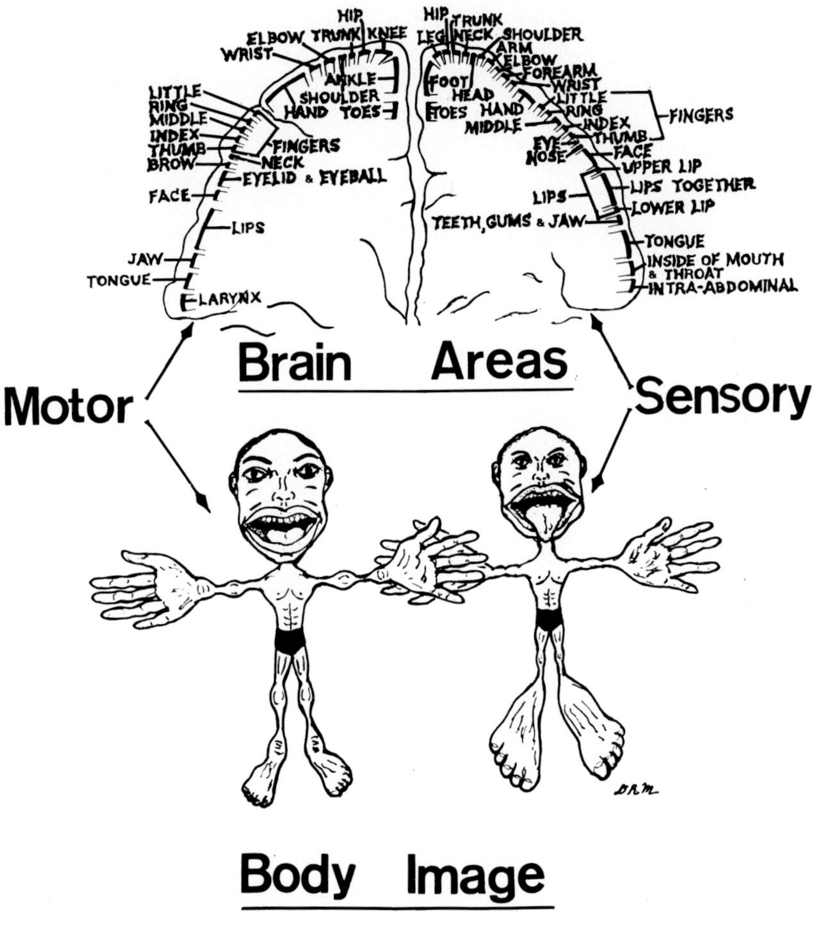

Figure 2-1.

many potential patients away from the office. However, even those who do go to the office have many fears. There have been a number of studies on physical and psychological dental fear-inducing agents (Box 2-4).

Box 2-4: The Frightened Tooth

Studies have been undertaken with respect to physiological and psychological changes occurring as the result of dental fear. Shannon and Isbel (1963) found that both the injection of a local anesthetic solution or the anticipation of the injection caused similar increases in serum corticosteroids. Venham and Quatrocelli (1977) showed that local anesthetic injections given to children over a period of six visits caused correspondingly more severe anxiety responses for each subsequent visit, as measured by heart rate change, anxiety level measurements, and independent ratings of cooperative behavior.

Messer's study (1977), using heart rate as an indicator, revealed that different patients reacted stressfully to different procedures. Lamb and Plant (1972) used anxiety-level questionnaires and showed that anxiety increased as treatment approached and drastically decreased after treatment. Edmonson and his co-workers (1972) found that patients with a specific dental phobia had higher levels of epinephrine before and during dental treatment, as compared to nonphobic controls.

Patients may become apprehensive at the first thought of going to the dentist (fear of the unknown or fear of pain). Even making the telephoned appointment can provoke anxiety. When the patient arrives at the dental office, the fear can begin in the reception room. It becomes intensified when the dental chair, dental unit, and instruments are seen. The specter of the dentist is often stressful to the apprehensive patient (Fig. 2-2). The touch of the explorer (the pick) or the blowing of air on the tooth are magnified to the frightened patient. But the worst fears are the fear of the needle and the drill.

Ordinarily, people do not willingly enter anxiety-laden or potentially painful situations. When certain people must face such a situation, disequilibrium occurs. They change their normal adult independent behavior into that of a helpless and dependent child (regressive behavior). This change occurs especially at the sight of the needle.

Some people actually panic at the sight of the needle. In some cases, it is the fear of the shot and the pain it causes. It is as if they were being stabbed by the dentist towering over them while they lie trapped in the confining dental chair. After the injection, there are fears about the numbness. "I can't talk. I can't stop drooling. I keep biting my lip. My face is swollen. I'll be numb for hours, but right now it's not numb enough. It

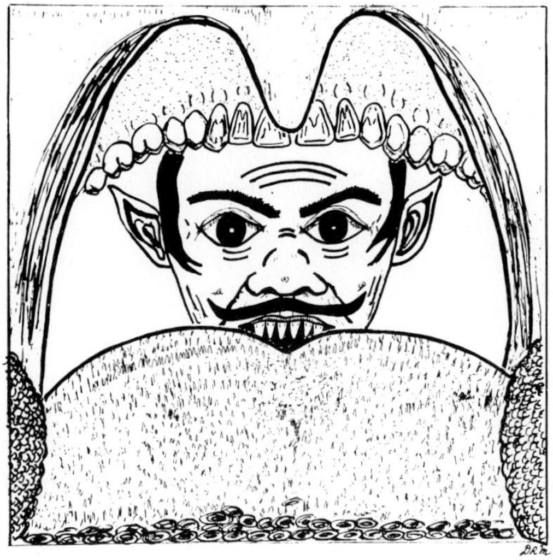

THE PATIENT'S VIEW
as "seen" from
inside of the mouth

Figure 2-2.

feels dead."

Fear of the drill is another well-known dental fear. Dental handpieces were formerly noisy, slow-speed, and ominous looking. The cutting bur appeared like a metalworker's tool bit. Part of the fear of the drill is connected to the similarity between dental drilling and the noisy, reverberating drill of the workman. The sound of the handpiece alone is stress inducing to many people.

Fear of extraction is another common fear. Apart from the Freudian fear of castration, fear of tooth loss is associated with fear of aging, fear of loss of beauty, and fear of mutilation. Having a nerve drilled into or removed is still the most frightening aspect of dentistry to the potential patient.

Other fears related to dental procedures are fear of radiation and fear of electric pulp testing. With the many recent pronouncements made about the dangers of x-rays, some patients have fears about the overuse of x-rays. With proper explanation, most of these fears can be overcome. Nevertheless, some patients adamantly refuse any x-rays, and this can be a source of serious conflict between a patient and a conscientious doctor. Explanation of what kind of response is expected when the electric pulp tester is employed is usually sufficient. However, fear of the potential electric shock causes some patients to refuse dental treatment if electric pulp testing is proposed.

One fear that is related to the fear of the unknown is the fear of not knowing what is wrong. For example, the patient may have severe oral pain or swelling and may fear that this is a symptom of a serious disease. Some patients may fear that they have cancer. This is especially true if the patient has a growth in the mouth. Studies show that women who postpone biopsy of breast tumors have a great fear of possible cancer and, therefore, avoid consulting the physician; the same may be true for oral lesions (Lazarus, 1966).

Other dentally related fears are fear of loss of control, fear of bleeding, fear of gagging or choking, and fear of bad treatment. Some conjectures patients might have with respect to the latter fear are "Will the wrong tooth be filled?" and "Will the tooth break?"

A final fear is the monetary fear. The character Babe in *Marathon Man* (Goldman, 1974) put it concisely, "Dentists raped you anyway; they charged a ton for maybe two minutes' work." As with any profession, that fear may occasionally be justified. More importantly, the primary fears, as noted earlier, are related to dental experiences, the psychosexual significance of the mouth, and the location of the self. How these fears can be overcome is discussed in Chapter 5. Table 2-I is a questionnaire to assess the patient's dental fears.

There are other stress-inducing reasons, apart from fear, that discourage people from going or returning to the dentist.

Table 2-I

QUESTIONNAIRE TO ASSESS PATIENT'S FEARS*

What is your feeling of fear? Rank the ten dental situations from the most to the least fearful. Then rate each dental situation from whether you feel very great to very little fear.

Dental Situation	*Rank*
Getting in the dental chair.	____

____	____	____	____	____
Very Great	Great	Average	Little	Very Little

Dentist tells you that you have bad teeth.	____
Dentist is giving you a shot.	____
Dentist is drilling your tooth.	____
Dentist squirts air into cavity.	____
Dentist puts probe into cavity.	____
Dentist is putting in the filling.	____
Dentist is doing root canal work.	____
Dentist is pulling your tooth.	____
Dentist is cleaning your teeth.	____

*Most studies have shown that the most fearful situations are root canal therapy, extractions, local anesthetic injections, and drilling.

Miscellaneous Causes of Patient Stress

Personal Space

Each person has his own *personal space*. This is based on *territoriality* (Ardrey, 1966; Morris, 1967), the theory that each individual has a personal "area" that he or she perceives as his own and must defend against outside invasion. The most intimate space ranges from actual physical contact to about 18 inches. Invasion of one's personal space can result in evasive, defensive, or aggressive action (Box 2-5).

Box 2-5: Too Close For Comfort

Two interesting studies relate to personal space. One study involved female students sitting in a library. It was found that when the female experimenter moved her chair within 1 foot of a female subject, 70 percent of the subjects approached in this manner moved away to less populated parts of the room. A second study involved fifteen prisoners, eight of whom had a history of aggressive behavior; the other seven were considered passive. The experimenter would move toward the center of the room where each subject took turns standing. The prisoner was to say "Stop" when the proximity of the experimenter made him feel uncomfortable. It was found that the aggressive prisoners demanded twice as much distance between themselves and the experimenter as did the passive prisoners (Baseheart, 1975).

Dentists repeatedly invade the patient's personal space, and this is quite upsetting to some patients. These patients may react by screaming, coughing, vomiting, fidgeting, talking, spitting out, or even being physically violent. As a result of the physical closeness between dentist and patient, some patients are upset by the patient's own bad breath (halitosis), the dentist's bad breath or body odor, and the touching by the dentist of the patient's head, face, shoulders, or other body parts.

Touching

Touching is considered to be a rather intimate, personal, sensual aspect of human contact. Touching in general is uncommon and not completely acceptable socially in the United States, particularly between two males. As far as touching various parts of the body, touching of the head is considered to be the most intrusive. Some patients, particularly men, become visibly upset when the dentist touches them in the head area (Box 2-6).

Box 2-6: The Not-So-Tender Touch

With respect to touching, one study reported the frequency of physical contacts between couples who were observed in cafes located in various countries. For example, the number of physical contacts made in some countries was as follows: San Juan, Puerto Rico, 180; Paris, France, 110; Gainesville,

Florida, 2; and London, England, 0. Specifically with the touching of various body parts, the study showed that the least amount of touching between men occurred in the head area. This finding also held for woman-to-woman contact (Baseheart, 1975).

Mannerisms and Habits

Apart from touch, there are other mannerisms and habits that annoy patients. Patients may be bothered by these behaviors of the dentist: He stares at patients; he picks his nose; he chews gum; he scratches his head or other body parts; he spits out regularly; he sings or whistles (usually in a monotone); he has a dry, hacking cough; he talks too much, too loudly, too quietly; or too little; and he pries into other people's business.

Unkempt Appearances

Patients can be "turned off" if the dentist or members of his staff are unkempt. Disagreeable aspects include dirty uniforms, dirty fingernails, scraggly hair, and unshaven faces.

The Physical Office

The physical attributes of the dental office can be stressful to the patients. Unclean, unsanitary offices are repellent. Patients dislike tasteless decor, unpleasant furnishings, stark or brilliant colors, uncomfortable furniture, loud music, musty odors, and oppressive humidity and temperatures (Box 2-7).

Box 2-7: Moods and Rooms

There are some interesting experiments involved with environmental factors. For example, the effects of an "ugly" room (looked like a disordered janitor's room) were compared to those of a "beautiful" room (carpeted, draped, etc.). The ugly room produced feelings of hostility, irritability, drowsiness, fatigue, monotony, and discomfort. The feelings produced by the beautiful room were energy, enjoyment, comfort, pleasure, and importance. Color has been associated with moods. Consider these: yellow, happiness and cheerfulness; blue, comfort and security; red, stimulation and excitement; brown and black, hostility, defiance, melancholia, dejection, despondence, and unhappiness.

In another study, high room temperatures were found to create more feelings of dislike between individuals than did lower, more moderate room temperatures. In still another study, it was found that placement of furniture can affect a person's reactions. When a desk interposed between doctor and patient, only 10 percent of the patients were judged to be at ease. When no desk acted as a barrier, 55 percent of the patients were judged to be at ease (Baseheart, 1975).

Treatment

There can be misunderstandings between dentist and patient because of failure to communicate; lack of rapport; and unsympathetic, abrupt, and inadequate or incomplete treatment. For example, a number of patients are now suing for nontreatment of periodontal disease or for extraction of a tooth when endodontic treatment should have been undertaken.

Finances

Inability to pay for dental services is an additional reason for patient stress. Often, the patient may be asked to accept a less than optimum treatment plan or even inferior and substandard treatment because he could not afford to pay for the better work.

Locus of Control

As discussed in Chapter 1, people whose locus of control is external may believe that "bad teeth" are genetic in origin and nothing can be done about it. These people may also believe that they have no control over their anxieties or fears for the same reasons. Conversely, those people whose locus of control is internal may believe something can be done and it is within their control, but are not sure how to go about gaining control. Methods of dealing with the patient stress-inducing factors in either event are discussed in Chapter 5.

Summary

Patient stress is related to dental fears and situations found in the dental office. Dental fears are widespread and are based on dental experiences, the psychosexual significance of the mouth, and the location of the self. The most severe dental fears are fear of the needle, fear of the drill, fear of nerve removal, and fear of extraction. Other stress-inducing reasons have to do with the appearance and behavior of the dentist and his staff, as well as with the dental office environment.

STRESS AND ORAL DISEASES

Introduction

Psychological, physical, and social stressors can result in distress, and repeated incidence of distress can lead to disease. In Chapter 4, the particular stress-related diseases and disorders to which dentists are prone are covered. In this section, consideration is given to the oral diseases and disorders that both patients and dentists can develop from repeated stressors.

Caries and Endodontic Diseases

The two principal groups of dental diseases are caries and periodontal diseases. One of the physiological effects during stress is decreased salivary secretion (xerostomia). Studies have shown that there is increased incidence of caries under conditions of reduced salivation. Other studies have also shown increased caries in animals that were stressed by repeated exercise as compared to immobilized animals (Protell et al., 1975).

When examining dental caries from a psychological standpoint, it has been observed that the periods of greatest dental caries in a person's life are generally adolescence and preadolescence. These are also the periods in a person's life when conditions for emotional or other psychological problems are most prevalent. The effects of repeated physical and psychological stressors that occur during these periods may predispose those individuals to caries, possibly as a consequence of diminished salivation and impaired immunological responses (related to excessive catecholamine and corticosteroid production).

If unchecked, caries can lead to pulpal and periapical diseases. Although only subjective descriptions can be relied upon, it appears that under conditions of stress, exacerbations of previously symptomless pulpitis and periapical pathoses can occur (Box 2-8). This often occurs under stressful conditions of increased altitude or barometric pressure (aerodontalgia). There may be some indirect causal relationship between stress and dental caries, pulpitis, and periapical diseases.

Box 2-8: Of Rats and Men

One of the authors (D.M.) had periapical surgery on an upper lateral incisor twenty-five years ago. At the present time, the tooth is symptomless, except during severe stressful situations when a painful toothache is experienced. When the stressful situation is resolved or is no longer perceived as such, the pain disappears. While there may be some periapical pathosis present, radiographically there is no evidence of this. One possible explanation is that there is an area of lowered resistance that predisposes to reaction under stress.

This condition could be related to the *weak organ theory* of psychosomatic disorders that states that under conditions of stress different people react in different organ systems to show clinical manifestations. Two examples are that blood pressure increases for some people and others have exacerbation of ulcers (Wolf, 1953).

A study by Stahl (1962) involves this concept. Gingival surgery was performed on rats that had been stressed nutritionally by being fed on a protein-deficient diet. The gingiva repaired after restoration of the protein to the diet. The rats were then again put on a protein-deficient diet, and even though surgery was not done a second time, the previously healed gingiva broke down a second time.

Periodontal Diseases

Of the various types of periodontal disease, the one with the closest association to stress is necrotizing ulcerative gingivitis (NUG; Vincent's disease). Several studies have shown that psychological stressors are important etiologic agents for NUG (Box 2-9).

Box 2-9: The Sympathetic Gums

Patients with NUG have been reported to be under more severe emotional strain than unaffected controls both in civilian and military activities. Studies of students have shown that they had increased incidence of NUG both before and during the taking of examinations. Crowding, as during military encounters, also seems to be a factor in the development of NUG. Another study showed that patients with NUG had statistically significant increased sympathetic nervous system responses, e.g. increased blood pressure, respiratory rate, and pupillary dilation, as compared to unaffected controls. Still other studies have shown significant relationships between sympathetic nervous system responses and high scores on anxiety-level tests for patients with gingivitis, periodontitis, and occlusal traumatism (Davis and Jenkins, 1962; DeMarco, 1976; Firestein, 1976; Giddon, 1966; Protell et al., 1975).

Clenching, Bruxism, and Myofascial Pain-Dysfunction Syndrome

Clenching involves intense, prolonged contact of opposing teeth without any grinding movement. Bruxing or gritting involves similar contact, but the teeth surfaces grind together. Both of these conditions are thought to be primarily a response to physical and psychological stressors, e.g. anger, and are correlated with latent aggression. Bruxism is generally found in angry, hostile, and dependent individuals. Repeated bruxing and clenching can lead to excessive tooth wear, pain of teeth on percussion, periodontal disease, fractured cusps, overdevelopment and spasms of masseter muscles, tension headaches, stiff neck, and the myofascial pain-dysfunction syndrome (MPDS). Many patients who develop MPDS have a history of moderate to severe depression.

Miscellaneous Oral Habits

Other oral habits related to stress are thumbsucking, lip-, cheek-, and nail-biting, and tongue thrusting. These deleterious habits can lead to malocclusions.

Tics

Tics are minor muscular twitches that have become habitual. The muscular movements are repetitive and usually purposeless. Tics may begin as voluntary responses to external or internal stimuli. However, after a period of time, they become habitual and involuntary. Tics probably are anxiety related and are expressions of psychological conflicts. They are more frequent in children. While tics can appear anywhere in the body, they are most common in the facial area. Those that are found in the mouth region are twitches of the lips and cheeks, continual clearing of the throat, "spitting out," and respiratory tics (as distinguished from allergies and respiratory ailments). The latter type includes uncontrollable coughing, sneezing, and hiccupping. Sometimes tics cease completely if they are ignored; other times they are chronic and may persist throughout life.

Aphthous and Herpetic Lesions

Recurrent aphthous ulcers are characterized by single or multiple ulcerous lesions (canker sores) that occur throughout the oral mucous membrane. Several studies have shown a close association between a history of emotional problems and development of aphthous ulcers (Francis, 1970; Greenfield and Fasciano, 1974; Protell et al., 1975; Scialfa, 1978; Ship, 1972). In animals given an auditory stressor, there was a higher incidence found of herpes stomatitis, as compared to nonstressed animals. Herpetic lesions in humans (cold sores) are also caused by the herpes simplex virus, and stress appears to be important in activation of the latent virus.

Miscellaneous Conditions

Other oral conditions shown to be related to psychological stressors are metallic taste, gagging, glossodynia (burning tongue), atypical facial neuralgia, angioneurotic edema, paresthesia, trismis, and cleft palate. Distortions in taste, such as metallic taste, have been reported to occur in mildly depressed individuals. It has been estimated that 90 percent of all gagging is psychological in origin. Many gaggers have fears of suffocation and of choking to death. Burning tongue may result from emotional conflicts or depression. Tongue thrusting is a habit that may be associated with anxiety. Atypical neuralgia often occurs in depressed post-menopausal females. Psychological stressors can precipitate angioneurotic edema, paresthesia, and trismis.

In animal experiments, it has been found that both hormones, such as cortisone and ACTH, and psychological stressors, e.g. noise of a buzzer, are capable of inducing a significantly higher incidence of cleft palates than in nonstressed controls.

Summary

Stress affects the oral cavity in many ways. The most common stress-related oral diseases are NUG, bruxism, myofascial pain-dysfunction syndrome, and recurrent aphthous ulcers. As a follow-up, the treatment of stress-related oral diseases is covered in Chapter 5. In Chapter 3, the dentist's stress is considered.

REFERENCES

Ardrey, R.: *The Territorial Imperative.* New York, Delta. Dell, 1966.

Baldwin, D. C., Jr.: An investigation of psychological and behavioral responses in dental extraction in children. *J Dent Res (Suppl. 6), 45:*1637, 1966.

Baseheart, J. R.: Nonverbal communication in the dentist-patient relationship. *J Prosthet Dent, 34:*4, 1975.

Bloomfield, J.: The initial interview. *Dent Clin North Am, 6:*601, 1962.

Borland, L. R.: Odontophobia — Inordinate fear of dental treatment. *Dent Clin North Am, 6:*683, 1962.

Cameron, N.: *Personality Development and Psychopathology.* Boston, Houghton Mifflin, 1963.

Cannistraci, A. J.: A method to control bruxism; biofeedback-assisted relaxation therapy. *J Am Soc Prev Dent, 6(12):*12, 1976.

Cassidy, J. E.: How to prevent dental phobia. *J Pedo, 1:*21, 1976.

Chue, P. W. Y.: Acute angioneurotic edema of the lips and tongue due to emotional stress. *Oral Surg, 41:*734, 1976.

Cinotti, W. R., Grieder, A., and Springob, H. K.: *Applied Psychology in Dentistry,* 2nd ed. St. Louis, Mosby, 1972, pp. 94-101.

Clarke, N. G. and Kardachi, B. J.: The treatment of myofascial pain-dysfunction syndrome using the biofeedback principle. *J Periodontol, 48:*643, 1977.

Corah, N. L. and Pantera, R. E.: Controlled study of psychologic stress in a dental procedure. *J Dent Res, 47:*154, 1968.

Cosgrove, D.: Sedation in dentistry. *Aust Dent J, 21:*128, 1976.

Crosby, J. F.: Theories of anxiety: A theoretical perspective. *Am J Psychoanal, 36:*237, 1976.

Davis, C. H. and Jenkins, C. D.: Mental stress and oral disease. *J Dent Res, 41:*1045, 1962.

DeMarco, T. J.: Periodontal emotional stress syndrome. *J Periodontol, 47:*67, 1976.

Edmonson, H. D., Roscoe, B., and Vickers, M. D.: Biochemical evidence of anxiety in dental patients. *Br Med J, 4:*7, 1972.

Eidelman, D.: A psychological aspect of dentistry. *Sven Tandlak Tidskr, 66:*393, 1973.

Epstein, S.: Psychological implications of anesthesia. *Dent Clin North Am, 6:*591, 1962.

Evans, F. J.: The placebo response in pain reduction. *Adv Neurol, 4:*289, 1974.

Firestein, S. K.: Patient anxiety and dental practice. *JADA, 93:*1180, 1976.

Francis, T.: Recurrent aphthous stomatitis and Behcet's disease. *Oral Surg, 30:*476, 1970.

Gale, E. N.: Fears of the dental situation. *J Dent Res, 51:*964, 1972.

Gale, E. N. and Ayer, W. A.: Treatment of dental phobias. *JADA, 73:*1304, 1969.

Gessel, A. H.: Electromyographic biofeedback and tricyclic antidepressants in myofascial pain-dysfunction syndrome: Psychological predictors of outcome. *JADA, 91:*1048, 1975.

Giddon, D. B.: Psychophysiology of the oral cavity. *J Dent Res (Suppl. 6), 45:*1627, 1966.

Greenfield, D. S. and Fasciano, R. W.: Oral ulcerative disease in young adults: Diagnosis and management. *J Am Coll Health Assoc, 23:*167, 1974.

Goldman, W.: *Marathon Man.* New York, Delacorte, 1974.

Guember, R. H.: Conquering dental fears. *Dent Manag, 17(11):*75, 1977a.

____ : The hidden faces of fear. *Dent Manag, 17(10):*73, 1977b.

Hall, C. S.: *A Primer of Freudian Psychology.* New York, World Publishing Co., 1954.

Hassett, J.: Why dentists are a pain in the mind. *Psychol Today, 11(8):*60, 1978.

Kirsch, A. J.: The psychiatric view of the mouth. *NY J Dent, 44:*117, 1974.

Kleinknecht, R. A., Klepac, R. K., and Alexander, L. D.: Origin and characteristics of fear of dentistry. *JADA, 86:*842, 1973.

Kordell, L.: *Lelord Kordell's Secrets for Staying Slim.* New York, Putnam, 1971.

Lader, M. and Marks, I.: *Clinical Anxiety.* New York, Grune, 1971.

Lamb, D. H. and Plant, R.: Patient anxiety in the dentist's office. *J Dent Res, 51:*986, 1972.

Laskin, D. M.: Editorial: The battered child. *J Oral Surg, 31:*903, 1973.

Lazarus, R. S.: Some principles of psychological stress and their relation to dentistry. *J Dent Res (Suppl. 6), 45:*1620, 1966.

____ : *Coping With Stress: Effects on Somatic Illness, Morale, and Social Functioning.* Read before the Symposium on Stress and Behavioral Medicine. New York, Dec. 3-4, 1977.

Lewis, T. M. and Law, D. B.: Investigation of certain autonomic responses of children to a specified dental stress. *JADA, 57:*769, 1958.

Messer, J. G.: Stress in dental patients undergoing routine procedures. *J Dent Res, 56:*362, 1977.

Morris, D.: *The Naked Ape: A Zoologist's Study of the Human Animal.* New York, McGraw, 1967.

Morse, D. R.: *Clinical Endodontology: A Comprehensive Guide to Diagnosis, Treatment and Prevention.* Springfield, Ill., Thomas, 1974, pp. 147, 150.

Protell, M. R., Krasner, J. D., and Fabrikant, B.: *Psychodynamics in Dental Practice.* Springfield, Ill., Thomas, 1975, pp. 3-41, 159-193.

Rosenberg, J. L.: Psychological evaluation of physical aspects of the dental office. *Dent Clin North Am, 6:*709, 1962.

Rosenzweig, S.: Psychological stress in cleft palate etiology. *J Dent Res (Suppl 6), 45:*1585, 1966.

Schaeffer, J. P.: *Morris' Human Anatomy,* 11th ed. New York, Blakiston, 1953, pp. 960-1055.

Schwartz, G. E.: *The Brain as a Health Care System: A Psychological Foundation for Stress and Behavioral Medicine.* Read before the Symposium on Stress and Behavioral Medicine. New York, Dec. 3-4, 1977.

Scialfa, C. T.: Electrical stimulation for the treatment of facial paresthesia and pain. *Dent Surv, 54(1):*42, 1978.

Shannon, I. L. and Isbel, G. M.: Stress in dental patients: Effect of local anesthetic procedures. *Dent Dig, 69:*459, 1963.

Ship, I. I.: Epidemiological aspects of recurrent aphthous ulcerations. *Oral Surg, 33:*400, 1972.

Sosnow, I.: The emotional significance of the loss of teeth. *Dent Clin North Am, 6:*637, 1962.

Stahl, S. S.: The effect of a protein-free diet on the healing of gingival wounds. *Arch Oral Biol, 7:*551, 1962.

Stricker, G. and Howitt, J. W.: Physiological recording during simulated dental appointments. *NY State Dent J, 31:*204, 1965.

Venham, L. and Quatrocelli, S.: The young child's response to repeated dental procedures. *J Dent Res, 56:*734, 1977.

Wolf, H. G.: *Stress and Disease.* Springfield, Ill., Thomas, 1953.

Zeldow, L. L.: Treating clenching and bruxing by habit change. *JADA, 93:*31, 1976.

Ziegler, H. P.: The sensual feel of food. *Psychol Today, 8(11):*62, 1975.

CHAPTER 3

THE DENTIST'S STRESS

Considered under the stress of being a dentist are (1) the kind of individual who becomes a dentist; (2) stress manifestations during schooling (predental, dental, and graduate levels); (3) the stress resulting from setting up a dental practice; (4) the stressors of dental practice, including patient, staff, and business management, the lack of exercise, companionship, and intellectual stimulation, and the routine nature of dental practice; (5) stresses outside of dental practice, covering social life, marital life, and investments; and (6) the stress of dental school and hospital teaching, embracing promotions, interpersonal relationships with staff, patients, other teachers and administrators, research problems, and publish-or-perish philosophy. A questionnaire to assess dentist stress is presented.

INTRODUCTION

HE was thirty-eight years old, a successful oral surgeon practicing in one of the metropolitan centers of the New South. It had been a busy Thursday; he spent the morning doing "general" in the "O.R." After a rushed lunch, he was back in the office for three I.V. cases, including a full-mouth extraction. At 4:45, the nurse escorted out the last patient. At 5:15, the receptionist left the office, after reminding the doctor about Friday's early morning appointment. As the door closed, he opened the top drawer of the I.V. cabinet. With calculated movements, he calmly loaded a syringe with meperidine. There was still some sunlight sifting through the treatment room window, so he closed the curtains. He took off his trousers, folded them neatly and placed them on the stool. Ever mindful of asepsis, he withdrew an alcohol sponge and placed it carefully on an area on the inside of his left thigh. Then, with deliberate speed, he emptied the contents of the syringe into the left femoral vein. Finally, he lay down on the operating table — never to awaken again.

This is a true story with only some of the details changed to maintain anonymity. Suicide and dentistry have been in the news recently. And though there is controversy over the true incidence of suicide by dentists, there is no doubt that dentistry can be a stressful occupation. In the remainder of this chapter, the various aspects of the stress of dentistry are considered.

The stress of dentistry is related to three major factors: (1) the type of individual who chooses dentistry as a career; (2) the competition of schooling; and (3) the choice within dentistry of engaging in general practice, a specialty, teaching, or administration.

DENTIST'S PERSONALITY AND SCHOOLING

The following topics are examined: (1) the profile of the student dentist; (2) predental training; (3) dental school; and (4) dental graduate school.

Profile of the Student Dentist

In discussing the dental student, the following are covered: (1) the family background; (2) the "frustrated physician syndrome"; (3) independence; (4) mechanical aptitude; and (5) miscellaneous conditions.

Family Background

There have been several studies concerned with the kind of individual who chooses dentistry (Protell et al., 1975). A review of what was learned could help clarify why dentists are prone to stress disorders. Recently, there has been an active recruitment into dentistry of low-income blacks, Hispanos, and females. The previous picture, however, of the entering dental student was that of a white, middle-class male. Surveys have shown that almost 10 percent of those who entered dentistry were sons (or daughters) of dentists, about 25 percent had parents who were professionals, and about 85 percent had fathers who were white-collar workers. Almost 70 percent of the entering students had college-educated fathers. With family backgrounds such as these, there is usually the family "push" for educational advancement and excellence. Minority students, who may be the first potential doctor in the family, might have an even greater family drive for them to succeed.

Frustrated Physician Syndrome

Are most dentists frustrated physicians? The evidence is unclear on this point. Formerly, it was much more difficult to get into and make it through medical schools than was the case for dental schools. Currently, however, it is almost as difficult to enter dental schools as it is to enter medical schools. For example, now one out of every 2.7 applicants is accepted into Temple University's dental school. In the medical school, it is one out of every 2.8 applicants. (Oddly enough, even though it is more difficult to get into veterinary school, dentists have never been considered frustrated veterinarians.)

It is more difficult in many ways to complete dental school than it is to complete medical school. For example, both manual dexterity and scientific acumen are necessary in dental school, whereas manual dexterity is not nearly as critical in medical school. Nevertheless, there are probably quite a few old-time practitioners who are frustrated physicians. This is not the usual case with the recent dental graduates. Few of the current entering dental students applied to medical school. It may be that they did not choose dentistry because they could not get into medical schools. Yet, the fear of rejection might have deterred some from applying (Box 3-1).

Box 3-1: The Age of Dentistry

In one survey, people who chose dentistry were asked to give their career preferences at various ages. At age ten, 17 percent of the students questioned listed medicine as a first choice, as opposed to only 5 percent picking dentistry as a first choice. In secondary schools, the students were about fifty-fifty in terms of first preference. In high school, 40 percent had dentistry listed as a first choice, as opposed to 20 percent, who listed medicine. In college, dentistry increased to 52 percent as medicine decreased to 17 percent. So, the further along students went in their education, the more they became oriented toward dentistry. Still, it is possible that the changing goals might have been related to the fact that their grades were not as high as thought necessary to get into medical school. Had they done better scholastically, a proportion of these students might have reserved medicine as a first choice (Sherlock and Morris, 1972).

Further evidence was the dental students' opinion of other professions. Eighty percent considered dentistry as more rewarding than law, university teaching, scientific research, pharmacy, and engineering (Sherlock and Morris, 1972). However, more than half of the students considered medicine to be more rewarding than dentistry. They rationalized their choice by stating that medicine was more difficult to enter and more demanding than dentistry (Box 3-2).

Box 3-2: The Unhappy Third

Recently, a comprehensive survey was conducted by *Dental Management* of the 1976 graduates of the University of Texas School of Dentistry at Houston. After one full year in practice, the respondents (about 50% of those solicited) were asked if they had to choose again, would they pick dentistry. About 30 percent stated that they would not choose dentistry. Most of them said they would opt for medicine: "I would choose a field in medicine like dermatology, which does not demand so much time and has financial rewards two and three times that of dentistry. And there is still more respect and prestige for the M.D." (Green, 1977).

Undoubtedly, dentistry is a second choice for some dentists. Studies have shown that those who enter a second-choice profession are more likely to show higher degrees of discontentment than those who aspired for and had reached their original goals (Sherlock and Morris, 1972).

Independence

Nevertheless, there are many students who picked dentistry over medicine as a first choice. They considered it better because of such things as (1) easier admission, (2) shorter training, (3) no evening or weekend practice, (4) less responsibility, (5) less competition for grades, (6) more prestige as a G.P. dentist than a general practitioner (hence, less need to become a specialist), and (7) being able to set the conditions and hours of one's own work. The students also considered dentistry as giving more opportunity than medicine for an individual to be self-employed and to get fees for services rather than from a salary. However, the one aspect of dentistry that was most favored may have the most stress-inducing potential; that is, most students gave the ability to be independent as their principal reason for choosing dentistry (Sherlock and Morris, 1972). While physicians have many daily contacts with other professionals at hospitals, the solo practitioner or independent dentist (still the prevalent practice) has few professional contacts. This could be a great source of discontent and distress.

Mechanical Aptitude

People who choose dentistry are believed to have special aptitude with their hands. It is thought that their interests, such as in sculpting and jewelry making, are associated with better than average manual dexterity. This mechanical ability is supposedly tested as part of the dental aptitude examination (DAT). But, not all dental students have "good hands," and this could be a source of frustration and failure while in dental school. It has been found that students who are clearly intellectually superior but lacking in mechanical skills have an extremely difficult time in dental school. Some inept dental students never graduate, and some who graduate eventually develop stress-related disorders. Others graduate, and their mechanical ineptitude follows them through their careers. In medicine, there are many more avenues for the intellectually gifted who happen to be inept manually. Not all physicians opt for surgery. Interestingly, those who choose dentistry for a career do not consider manual dexterity to be the most important reason for entering dentistry (Sherlock and Morris, 1972). Unfortunately, they find the reverse to be true while in dental school, i.e. the school's main objective is to produce excellent technicians, and in their dental practice. The disparity between the students' interpretation of the importance of manual dexterity and its real focus could become a severe stress-inducing factor.

Miscellaneous Considerations

Almost 80 percent of the dental students interviewed in one survey stated that they chose dentistry because they expected to earn a higher income and aspired to a standard of living greater than that of their parents (Sherlock and Morris, 1972). This could also be a source of frustration if these goals are not achieved.

Most dental students stated that they did not enter dentistry for altruistic reasons but rather to be "successful" in life (defined as the chance to make money and gain prestige) and to be independent. People choosing dentistry tend to be pragmatic rather than idealistic. They are characterized as materialistic, utilitarian, and conservative. What is not clear is whether they develop these attitudes after exposure to the "real life" of dentistry or if they had these attitudes throughout most of their lives. At any rate, a practical individual could become distressed if his materialistic goals were not realized.

One motivational factor for future dentists is frequent exposure to dentists in childhood. This could be a source of later stress if the practice of dentistry does not live up to the student's preconceived notions of dentistry.

A final characteristic attributable to some potential dentists is *subliminal aggression.* If there are some dentists who have this failing, they might be less stressed than others, since these dentists would have a chance to release their aggressive tendencies via injecting, drilling, and extracting. Fortunately, it is more likely that most potential dentists are kind, gentle, and considerate — and the fact that some patients consider dentists to be sadistic would be a great source of distress to these dentists.

Predental Training

As indicated earlier, some people choose dentistry for a career while still in elementary school. If they do not elect dentistry, they favor medicine. So, they begin the competitive cycle and work hard to obtain A's. By the time they have reached high school, they have heard from the grapevine that to get into a prestige college is very important, i.e. because it is easier to get into professional school from a top-ranked university or college. In addition, in order to get into a "good" school one needs extracurricular activities as well as high grades. (Presumably this assures the admissions committee that the applicant is "well rounded.") So, there is a "mad rush" into such activities as athletics, theater, student newspapers, student government, and choral groups. In addition, the A's must still be obtained — and are neurotically pursued. One important side effect of this striving is that practically no time remains for simple relaxation.

Once the student gets into college, the competition intensifies. Premed and predental students take the same courses, and although the competition is stiffer to get into medical schools, the predental students still feel it. Under pressure of this kind, students use all methods, including cheating and threats to teachers, to get high grades. In many cases, the guilt and stress exact a higher price than the return. Often, the knowledge of the subject is only incidental. There are times when the teachers add to this pressure (Box 3-3).

Also, to be outstanding in collegiate extracurricular activities, e.g. class president, newspaper editor, or football hero, is considered advantageous. In addition to the "paper chase," the intense competition can cause serious distress. In fact, at one Ivy League school there has been an average of one suicide per year. Statistics indicate that suicide is the second leading cause of college-related deaths (accidents are first, but some may be disguised suicide). Finally, some students do get into professional school. Instead of decreasing, the pressures increase.

Box 3-3: The A-B Reverse Twist

> One of the authors (D.M.) took an embryology course in his senior year in college. His grades were in the 90's. The course instructor had a policy of only giving three A's in a class, regardless of the students' achievements. Since D.M. already had been accepted into dental school, he was informed by the professor that while an A would reflect his achievement, he was going to get a B. The professor intended to give the A (that rightfully belonged to D.M.) to a premed student who could use the grade to get into medical school. In those days, student protest usually went unheeded. D. M.'s appeals to reason and fairness were futile. The incident was quite upsetting and, after all these years, still has not been forgotten.

Dental School

The stress-inducing factors of dental school are related to (1) the students, (2) the curriculum, (3) the teaching staff, (4) the patients, (5) the administration, and (6) the physical facilities of the school. The personality of the entering student has already been discussed. In the first two years of dental school, there is a heavy concentration of basic sciences, along with the introduction of preclinical courses. The intense competition for grades carries over into dental school. It used to be that about 85 percent of dental students stayed in general practice upon graduation (Sherlock and Morris, 1972). Today, more students progress to specialty training. One of the prime considerations for acceptance into specialty programs is academic performance while in undergraduate dental school. (Once again, the students are addressed as freshman and sophomore.) Thus, there is some rationale for the competition for grades. Even without that influence, the competition between students is used by some dental school instructors and departments as a way to spur high performance. Conversely, the relatively low level of cooperation among dental students may be a reflection of the independent character of their personalities.

A consequence of the intense competition for grades that often begins in elementary school is found in the forced isolation of the average dental student. As a result, he is often immature emotionally, sexually, and professionally and may suffer bouts of anxiety. There may be an intense fear of failing, separate from the need to achieve, which reinforces the maladaptive behavior of avoiding study by the dental students. Thus, this vicious cycle greatly increases the chances of failure and increases stress. Of course, not all students react this way. In some cases, students operate well under pressure, and threat of failure motivates and facilitates high performance in such students.

Studies have shown that dental students' ethics decline from the first to fourth years. Cynicism increases, especially in the last two years (Sherlock and Morris, 1972). Idealistic students caught in this turmoil may become severely stressed. One survey of three California dental schools found that by the time they were seniors, most dental students considered the important aspects of dentistry to be autonomy, prestige, social mobility, and income rather than professional service, altruism, or technical competence (Sherlock and Morris, 1972). Again, this could be a source of conflict and anxiety to dental students who went into school with other ideals.

Another source of potential distress to the student is the disproportionate amount of time they spend in the basic sciences on material they believe to be irrelevant. The lack of relevancy attitude is based on (1) the material itself; (2) the teacher's inability to communicate other than abstractly (especially if the courses are taught by pure-science professors); and (3) the students' (and later, practitioners') unwillingness to try to integrate clinical findings with basic science knowledge. It is a source of stress when dental students receive their basic sciences courses with medical students. Here, there is even less reference to clinical dentistry, and often the dental students are treated as inferiors.

Cheating is rampant in some schools, and many of the better students become distressed because of it. They also may be chastised by their peers if they fail to share this norm.

The undue emphasis in some schools on mechanical skills can certainly be a source of frustration. Margins must be perfect, root canal fillings must be flush with the apex, and restorations must have mirrorlike finishes. Anything short of these ideals usually results in criticism (often in front of the patient) or poor grades. Although it is important that standards are set, unfortunately, the concept of perfection follows many dentists throughout their lives.

Emphasis on mechanics in many schools is accompanied by de-emphasis on research and teacher training. This can only add to the students' feeling that dentistry is mechanically oriented. Students interested in research and teaching may find it difficult to achieve their goals. Even if they eventually pursue their interests, they may become frustrated with the mechanical skill being emphasized in dental schools.

Part of dental school stress is related to the teachers. Many dental instructors have had no teacher training. Until recently, there has been a high proportion of military service retirees, dental practice dropouts, and part-time instructors. Some teachers let out their frustrations on the students. The teacher-student transaction tended to be, "I'm O.K., you're not O.K." Recently, with better salaries and fringe benefits available, dentistry is attracting teachers with more commitment and preparation. However, with each dental department convinced of the relative importance of its curriculum and area, many students feel overburdened with assignments. Some of the experienced teachers believe that stress is an important part of the professional training. The belief is that if the student cannot manage a moderately stressful situation in school, he will not be able to handle the real stress that occurs in practice. Unfortunately, some students "crack" from the overemphasis placed by some instructors on this approach. Many respondents from the Houston dental school survey felt that "the unreasonable minutia and needless 'brow beatings' have generated long-lasting feelings of incompetence" (Green, 1977).

One can get an idea of how students feel about some of their instructors by reading the walls of the dental school toilet stalls, i.e. graffiti. This is also a place for some of the students to release their frustrations and anxieties.

Another aspect of dental student distress is related to patients. Dental students generally get to see their first patient in the third year (sooner in some schools) and take on the role ordinarily found in outside practice. In contradistinction, in medicine, the practice-type patient-doctor relationship is generally not seen until internship or residency. In one survey, it was found that dental students perceive themselves as entering a profession that has an unfavorable public image (Protell et al., 1975). This feeling is enlarged by the dental student-patient encounters in the dental school clinics. Although some patients are relaxed in the dental chair, many patients manifest apprehension or have covert feelings of dread. This anxiety is readily transferred to the dental students.

Some graduates go into the military service or public health because they feel the lack of capability to manage independent private practice. It may take as long as five years before some graduates feel ready to risk private practice.

Another source of student stress is financial. The cost of dental education is becoming astronomical, and many students are forced to work. One study found that students' attitudes toward finances changed in the senior year (Sherlock and Morris, 1972). Many dental student seniors thought of themselves as craftsmen, salesmen, businessmen, and entrepreneurs (predominantly related to financial aspect of practice), rather than as health educators or researchers. Again, these changing values could be a source of stress to some students.

Many students are forced to provide family support, and this is another source of stress. One survey found that by the senior year, three out of five students were married, and many had families (Protell et al., 1975). Often, wives were working. The arrangement of full-time students, working wives, and dependent children could add marital stressors to the other factors. Some students may want to go into specialization, but do not because of family ties and lack of money. They either borrow a lot of money to open a practice (and then worry about whether they will be able to pay it back), or they go into the military service or public health.

During the senior year, dental students face yet another stress-inducing obstacle, that is, the taking of state board examinations. There is intense competition to get suitable patients, and the actual taking of the exam is one of the most stressful times in the dental student's or dentist's life.

If the administration is inflexible, curriculum often remains fixed, instructors and teaching methods stay static, and facilities may become dreary places in which to work. Working in run-down open clinics with antiquated equipment can be disheartening for even the best student. Fortunately, most administrators are flexible and many schools are undergoing creative change.

At any rate, most students are graduated and then, contrary to these students' expectations, heavy stress begins.

Dental Graduate School

Some students do not enter private practice immediately but opt for a specialty. Others practice for a time and then apply to a graduate program. Many of the stressors of graduate training are similar to those found in undergraduate dental school. An additional source of distress is the fact that many students are older and have already practiced as dentists. To go from being a money-earning dentist to a money-spending student again can be quite distressing to some. Another aspect of graduate school training is the small size of the graduate class. The protection afforded through maintenance of a low profile in undergraduate dental school with its large student body is no longer possible. Individual performance is closely observed, and there is the greater possibility of personality clashes.

DENTAL PRACTICE

Introduction

The stress of dental practice is related to (1) setting up practice; (2) the kind of training received; (3) patients' feelings; (4) responsibility; (5) competition for patients; (6) office management; (7) independence; (8) isolation; (9) finances; (10) the dental area of specialization; (11) the mechanics of practice; (12) drugs; (13) type of practice; (14) social considerations; and (15) family life.

In the Beginning

Setting up a dental practice is a stressful time for the new practitioner. Suddenly thrust into the real world from the protected environment of dental school, he must now concern himself with getting started in practice. Stressors associated with setting up practice are (1) finding a location both to practice and to live; (2) obtaining the money for purchasing of home, office, equipment, and supplies; (3) selecting equipment; (4) hiring staff; (5) purchasing insurance; and (6) meeting prospective patients. An ADA estimate (1977) is that the average dental student is $13,000 in debt upon graduating and spends $40,000 to $50,000 to set up a practice.

Rather than opening his own practice, the recent graduate may become associated with an established practitioner. However, here also there may be stress that is related to —

1. Different philosophies and techniques of the two doctors
2. Personal relationships with the doctor and his staff
3. Lack of personal control of practice

Overtrained Dentists

While in dental school, dentists are exposed to idealized dentistry calling for treatments such as porcelain restorations, precision attachments, molar endodontics, and refined periodontal procedures. Yet, in the early years of a new practice, especially in a developing suburb, patients delay or forego the more expensive procedures. Therefore, the fledgling dentist spends most of his day in cleaning, filling, and pulling. This can generate feelings of guilt because the dentist is not practicing ideal dentistry as he was taught to do in dental school.

When the beginning dentist gets beyond the "drilling-filling-billing" stage, he is often forced to compromise because of fees. So, although he believes the patient needs a fixed bridge, he makes a removable partial, or he extracts a tooth rather than performing endodontics. Compromise engenders frustration.

The high cost of dentistry can also engender guilt feelings in the dentist. He may be torn between (1) lowering his fees to accommodate patients, (2) maintaining his fees to keep competitive with the other dentists in the area, and (3) raising his fees commensurate with providing quality dentistry. Sometimes "better" dentistry is accepted by patients, but only after much time spent selling. Dentists may become stressed because they have to sell a service that is often in the patient's best interest.

When the dentist does get a chance to do high-quality, exacting procedures, he gets upset when failures occur or less than "perfect" results are achieved. Dentists tend to be perfectionists either innately or as a result of their dental school training. Thus, when less than ideal results are obtained, dentists often blame themselves, even though there is no fault of their own. Lack of patient cooperation or imperfect laboratory procedures may have contributed to the outcomes. Fear of failure or actual failure is associated with self-blame. Self-blame is destructive and leads to distress and disease.

It has been said that "physicians bury their mistakes" and "dentists' mistakes come back to haunt them." Such statements may be only partially true, but some dentists are distressed by them.

Little of the knowledge gained in fulfilling the basic science requirements of dental training is found relevant or useful by the practitioner in the early stages of clinical practice. Some anxieties are associated with feelings of being overprepared for the tasks at hand.

Undertrained Dentists

In dental school, emphasis is placed on restorative dentistry and prosthodontics. Less time is spent on orthodontics, oral surgery, and endodontics. As mentioned earlier, in the building phase of most practices, routine restorations and simple extractions are the principal procedures performed. Hence, the budding practitioner may not have the capability that an orthodontist, oral surgeon, or endodontist has, especially for difficult cases. A lot of mental anguish can be built up in attempting to remove an impacted third molar or attempting instrumentation in a calcified root canal. Therefore, general dentists should learn early in their careers to refer difficult cases to specialists. Physicians are usually more inclined than dentists to refer complex or problem cases to other physicians and they do not consider themselves less capable because of it. However, the dentist should not become a "referral station," because constantly doing procedures such as occlusal or interproximal amalgams is monotonous.

Also related to the type of procedures performed is the dentist's personal preference. Many dentists do procedures they detest either because it is expected of them, or they want the income. However, it would be kinder to a practitioner's mental state if he referred endo- or pedodontics cases if those kinds of procedures or patients disturbed his equilibrium.

Another aspect of undertraining or inadequate preparation is the management of the severe office emergency. Formerly, dental schools gave minor consideration to the diagnosis and treatment of the medical emergency patient. Now, all dental schools give adequate training in office emergency procedures, but most dentists rarely see a true emergency, e.g. coronary occlusion, cerebral stroke, or insulin shock. Thus, they may be unprepared to handle such a reaction. Dentists worry about the possibility, and some poorly managed emergencies occur. In comparison, most physicians often deal with medical emergencies in their offices or in the hospital, so they are well prepared. Periodic rehearsals by dentists with their staff could help decrease this source of stress.

Patient Fear and Hate

Dentists first encounter patients' fears while in dental school.

Notwithstanding that fact, dental school patients generally tolerate the clinical situation better than patients consulting private dentists. This is probably related to the lower fees the patients pay and the longer time that they are seen by the students. Students get a chance to know their patients because of the nature of dental education, which by necessity prolongs the time required for each procedure. In private practice, fear is greater and pain more intense, at least in the perception of patients. Patients who pay more expect more, and as a result, their complaints often are magnified. Constantly hearing about pain and fears traumatizes even a well-insulated dentist.

It is uncanny that the dentist is always depicted as causing pain (in contrast to the image of the physician, who is seen as relieving pain). On occasion, dentists inflict pain in the course of treatment. Sometimes, the inferior alveolar injection is not completely successful. At times, a painful intrapulpal injection must be done. Causing pain may add to the guilt of the compassionate dentist.

Not only is there fear, but hate may be transferred to the dentist. Every dentist hears remarks such as "I hate the dentist," "I hate going to the dentist," "I'd like you if you weren't a dentist," and "I'd rather have a baby than go to the dentist." This too takes its toll.

Responsibility

Dealing with patients carries responsibility. This is true for all health professionals. Perhaps it is greatest for the physician, who deals with life-and-death situations. But, if one is a conscientious dental practitioner, the weight of responsibility can be a heavy burden, and severe distress can result. The responsibility is so all-encompassing for some that they never even take a vacation because of the fear of not knowing who will take care of their patients while they are away. On the other hand, a few dentists actually thrive on responsibility and may seek out difficult cases.

Competition for Patients

Some dentists do not take vacations and become overly solicitous to patients for other reasons, such as fear of the loss of patients and worry that the practice will fall apart. This can be a serious consideration if a dentist practices in an area that is saturated with dentists or if the economy happens to be on a downswing.

Office Management

By the time dental students are seniors, they realize that dentistry is a business, and administration of the office is very important. This is another source of stress, since they are ill prepared to face the managerial problems of the dental office.

Ordering equipment and supplies, training and working with staff, dealing with the laboratory and dental salesmen, regulating the schedule, balancing the books, analyzing insurance forms, paying bills, working on overdue accounts — all of these should not be the dentist's responsibility, and yet all too often they are. Another stressful circumstance with effects that may last for years is the receipt of a malpractice action. Whether warranted or not, the fact that one is being sued can "gnaw internally" and cause considerable distress (Wolfe, 1978).

There is also the problem of time utilization. Trying to fit in emergencies in an already crowded schedule can be nerve racking. Also, it is unnerving when the dentist falls short of time, and patients are waiting impatiently in the reception room. In contrast, physicians can arrange to see several people in the same time slot. Not only can each patient wait in a different room, but the patients receive a certain amount of preparatory treatment by the nurses. It is not expeditious for a dentist to work on two or three patients simultaneously. When he attempts this, he works "on roller skates" and often finds that the quality of his work suffers, and his stress increases.

Time pressure is often self-inflicted. Dentists decide that they must do a certain amount of work in an alloted time. Many dentists think, "I have to make 'X' amount of dollars per hour to be productive." The whole problem of time sharing is one of the most exacting sources of stress in the dental office.

Dentists have enough trouble conducting their own businesses. Sadly, all too many become involved in outside investments. Many dentists develop ulcers because of stock losses. Land deals, cattle, oil wells, and restaurant chains have contributed considerably to dentists' hypertensive states.

Finances

Money begets money which begets stress which begets money, ad infinitum. The dentist makes a good living, buys a nice house, a "classy" car and fine clothes and takes "fancy" vacations. In addition, then, if he is married, he and his wife want more. So he works harder, sees more patients, keeps longer hours, or charges higher fees in order to make more money. This vicious cycle can only lead to breakdown.

Independence and Isolation

As mentioned previously, the solo practice is still the principal type of dental practice. Dentists practicing alone have little opportunity to communicate with other professionals. They cannot share their professional problems or personal anxieties (Box 3-4).

Box 3-4: Fear Loves Company

In a series of classic experiments to study the effects of fear on affiliative behavior, Stanley Schachter (1959) compared highly fearful women who expected intense shock with low-fear women who expected mild shock. Schachter found that highly fearful subjects chose to wait with one another significantly more often than did the women who had little cause for alarm. Stress, then, is one condition that increases affiliative behavior. Dentists who are under stress in solo practice have little opportunity to seek out other professionals, and if they are highly fearful individuals, they would have problems in managing their fears.

Dentists often have to make decisions on their own while they are alone. Studies have shown that decision making provokes many psychological stressors, including frustration, irritability, anxiety, fear, pride, and joy (Miller, 1977). Being unsure of decisions can cause the dentist to turn inward and use potentially negative coping methods, such as suppression, emotional insulation, and rationalization (*see* Chap. 6). Loneliness also often precipitates depression.

In addition, many dentists practice at the same location with the same equipment and the same staff year after year. Monotony engenders stress. In comparison, physicians have more of an opportunity to communicate with colleagues and others because of their hospital and clinic affiliations.

Living dentistry without respite can add to the stress potential. When dentists interact, far too often they criticize each other's work. Studies have shown that this behavior begins in dental school (Sherlock and Morris, 1972). At social gatherings, dentists too often sit with other dentists and "talk shop," giving outsiders the impression that dentists are narrow and pedestrian.

If dentists become involved in multiple practices with colleagues and many auxiliaries, other stressors that pertain to personalities and interpersonal and working relationships become evident.

The Dental Area

Dentists work in an enclosed area in proximity to their patients for extended periods of time. This arrangement can interfere with both the dentist's and patient's personal spaces. The constant close contact can be stressful to both. Dentists tend to see mouths rather than people (Fig. 3-1), and patients tend to see an ogre rather than a doctor (*see* Fig. 2-2). Patients would like their dentists to see them as more than teeth with a body attached. The close contact may be felt as intimate and takes on sexual significance in terms of the psychosexual significance of the oral cavity.

The physical arrangement can be stressful in another way. There are some patients who come to the dentist, recline on the contoured chair — much as on a psychiatrist's couch — and present their innermost problems, fully expecting empathetic listening, if not psychological counseling. This onus on the dentist, who is ill prepared for this role, produces stress.

Continual contact, with numerous patients, can cause physical stressors to affect the dentist. These include infective mi-

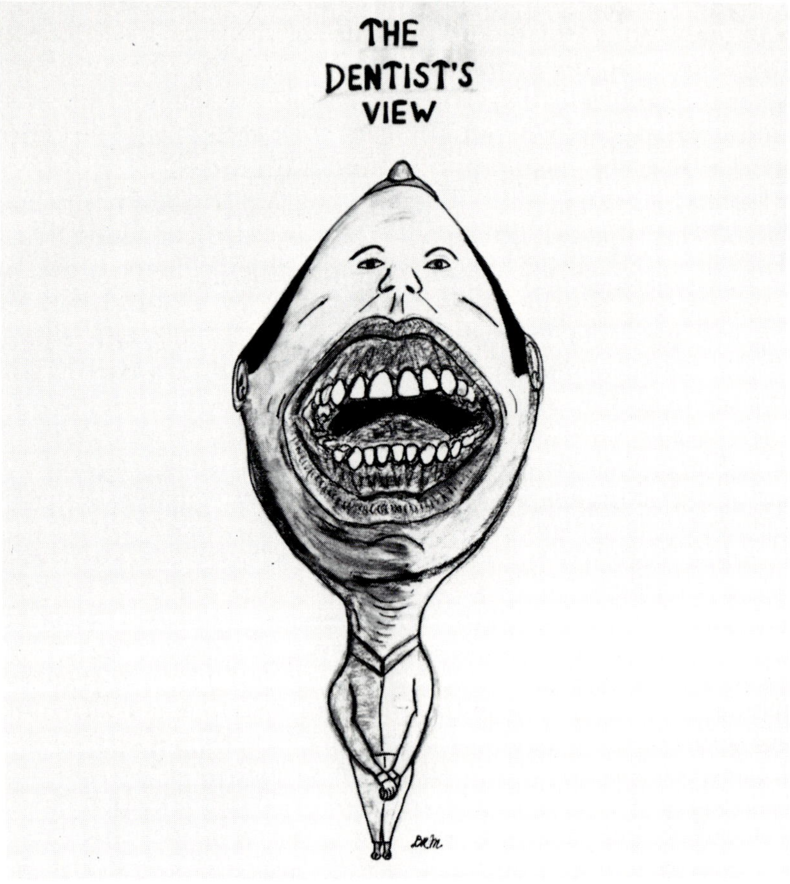

Figure 3-1.

croorganisms (hepatitis and venereal diseases) and potentially toxic gases (nitrous oxide) and chemicals (mercury). Too much sitting results in physical inactivity and does not allow for adequate exercise. Unrelieved standing affects circulation and fosters varicosities. Continuous bending over patients results in kyphosis, lordosis, and scoliosis, i.e. back problems, and internal organ disorders. A recent survey by the Pierre Fauchard Academy found that one out of every three dentists has a back malady (Foley, 1977).

The average dental treatment room can be more than confining. The typical small-sized room (on the average, 8-by-10 feet) replete with the dental armamentarium and without any distractive appointments can be an additional stress factor.

There are other physical stressors related to the work area. Noise can cause permanent hearing damage (the higher frequencies are particularly affected), and there is a constant source of destructive noise coming from both the low- and high-speed handpieces (Box 3-5).

Box 3-5: The Ill Drill

Tests conducted at Loyola University have shown that high-speed handpiece noise adversely affects the hearing of the operator. Other deleterious responses found were increased blood pressure, decreased hand reflex time, and an increase in the number of eye-hand coordination errors (Foley, 1977).

Lighting is another problem. Constantly going from a well-lit area (oral cavity) to less illuminated areas causes eyestrain. The noxious odors of the dental office can be offensive and sickening to both dentist and patient.

Another problem may arise for the solo practitioner who works with one assistant. In this situation, the dentist and assistant work together as a team for many hours each day. Depending upon the mutual attraction, relationships can develop that may extend outside of the office. The consequences may be counterproductive and destructive to dentist, assistant, and any extant spouses (Rosenbaum, 1978).

The Mechanics

Dentists have to perform meticulous manipulative movements in a small area for most of the working day. They usually work on conscious and vigilant patients who often react negatively. The dentist must be as "sharp" at 5 PM as he was at 9 AM. During treatment, social intercourse between dentist and patient is often one-way, with staccato instructions such as "Open," "Close," "Spit out," and "Open wider." In contrast, physicians spend a large part of their office day in talking, examining, and writing prescriptions. When they do perform surgical procedures, they are generally done in a hospital setting, and the patient is under general anesthesia and is passive. So, by the nature of his work, the dentist probably is confronted by more physical and psychological stressors than is a physician (Box 3-6).

Box 3-6: The Tired Dentist

> In the survey at the University of Texas at Houston dental school, approximately 25 percent of the respondents of the class of 1976 admitted to being fatigued by the end of the day. The majority attributed the exhaustion to the hard physical work of being a dentist, but they also felt that their fatigue was a consequence of the mental concentration inherent in dental practice (Green, 1977).

Drugs

Dentists have easy accessibility to drugs. They also know how effective tranquilizers, barbiturates, sedatives, and nitrous oxide can be to overcome apprehension. Thus, it is easy to use these drugs on themselves when trouble is imminent. Unfortunately, the drugs may cause an addiction or even provide the vehicle for attempting suicide.

The Fragmentation of Dentistry

Another potential source of stress that can affect the practicing dentist is the possible fragmentation of dentistry. There are (1) pro- and antifluoridationist dentists; (2) pro- and anti-expanded function of auxiliaries dentists; (3) pro- and antidenturists; (4) pro- and anti-third-party dentists; and (5) pro- and anti-mandatory peer review dentists. If fluoride were to be completely successful, the dentist's role and income might change and decrease. The same could be said for increased utilization of auxiliaries and denturists. With more third-party arrangements, many dentists feel that they are losing control of the practice of dentistry.

Further potential fragmentation is the problem that dentists have in certain hospitals in regard to lack of privileges and authority in contrast to the status enjoyed by physicians. The purported inferiority complex of the dental profession vis-à-vis the medical profession could feed to the level of the individual dentist and be a source of stress.

The dental media sometimes reinforces these stressors by constantly reminding the dentist about (1) the terrible problems of peer review, denturism, third-party dentistry, and antifluoridationists; (2) unfair treatment by the medical profession; and (3) shortage or surplus of dentists (depending upon which statistics are read). Perhaps, if dentists read with more critical judgment, this might decrease their neuroses, and their individual stress levels would decline.

The Specialties

When a dentist enters a specialty, he generally earns a higher income than a general practitioner. However, the trade off is doing more of the same procedures, with increased monotony. This is especially true in specialties such as endodontics and oral surgery (exodontia). Yet, this source of potential distress is not unique to dentistry; it also exists in medicine.

Different specialties present singular problems. In orthodontics, the longtime relationship is with children. In perio- and prosthodontics, there are prolonged relationships with adult and aged patients. In oral surgery and endodontics, there are short-term relationships. Both short- and long-term relationships can be stressful to particular individuals.

Other specialty-related problems are (1) for prosthodontists, partial dependence upon laboratory technicians; and (2) for periodontists, treating patients who come in without pain and subsequently develop pain (hypersensitive dentin and cementum).

Also, the kind of patient consulting the practitioner presents special problems. Pedodontists see frightened children; endodontists and oral surgeons see frightened adults. These specialists have to be well prepared to cope with these kinds of patients. Prostho- and periodontists may see many change-of-life patients who often have psychological "hang-ups," and this can be distressful to those specialists.

Another potential stressor of specialty practice is status. In order to advance, it is essential to take board examinations. These examinations are difficult and stressful for even the best-prepared candidates.

The Social Aspect

In trying to build a practice, whether it is general or a specialty, it is usually necessary for the dentist to attend meetings, give lectures, have parties, and generally become socially active. General dentists have to cater to patients; specialists have to cater to both patients and referring dentists. These obligations could be discomforting for the shy, introverted dentist and could be annoying to the outgoing, extroverted person. Dentists also have to worry about visibility. They concern themselves with such things as "Should I buy a 'Caddy' or a 'Mercedes'?" "What will the patients think?" or "Can I be seen mowing the lawn or repairing the roof?"

Family Life

In common with many professionals, dentists often take their problems home with them. The spouse may have problems of his or her own. This conflict can produce strife and often creates divorce.

Often, wives work while their husbands are going through school and during the early stages of the developing practice. When the husband begins to earn a good living, the wife may feel that she is no longer needed (as she was needed during the dental school years). This change in circumstance also precipitates strife. Some wives work in the dental office. Even considering the tax advantages, constant nearness without respite both in and out of the office can be disturbing to both partners. There is also tax advantage in the office-home combination. The disadvantage lies in having the problems of family and children spill over into the office.

Another factor related to the family and social pressures is the location of the dental practice. One study showed that major illnesses and depression had a much lower incidence in the southern as compared to the eastern United States (Redmond, 1977a). The South has traditionally been considered to have a more relaxed life-style, and this seems to affect the incidence of stress-related disorders in dentistry. City living versus suburban or country living is another stress-related factor. City living is generally considered to be more stressful.

DENTAL TEACHING

Introduction

The stress of teaching results from (1) interrelationships with staff, patients, other teachers, and administrators; (2) tenure and promotions; (3) salary; (4) teaching; (5) publish-or-perish philosophy; and (6) research problems.

Interrelationships

A dental school reminds one of a small town: Everybody is aware of everyone else's business. To be successful in teaching, one has to be able to get along with the departmental chairman, other teachers, the administrators, the staff, the students, and the patients. This is an imposing task, especially for the dentist who treasures his independence. Dentists who are used to being the boss and running a solo practice may find it distressing to be in a situation where they have to cater to others. As with other businesses, petty jealousies are part of the teaching atmosphere. All of these factors have special significance in a dental school providing professional training and tend to amplify the stressors generally found in an undergraduate college.

Tenure, Promotions, and Salary

Security is one of the reasons why dentists enter teaching. To achieve security, it is necessary to obtain tenure. To make more money, promotions are necessary. The stated criteria for tenure and promotion are outstanding teaching, research, and community service. In actual practice, it is also necessary to follow orders and not assert the independence that so many dental students listed as a reason for entering dentistry in the first place. Thus, some dentists find it difficult to adjust to teaching in such an environment.

Even with the granting of tenure and obtaining promotions, the financial remunerations of teaching fall far short of what can be achieved in private practice. The thought of this can be a persistent irritant to the dedicated teacher and perhaps more so to the teacher's spouse.

Teaching

Teaching requires (1) hours of preparation, (2) designing exams, (3) grading exams, (4) having to answer to students for the exams, (5) counseling students, (6) doing administrative duties, (7) reviewing and grading research papers, (8) serving on various school committees, and (9) in a dental school, checking off clinical cases. (This is the instructor's principal responsibility in some clinical departments.) These diverse roles of the teacher can be stress inducing at particular times. One particular example stands out. In the clinic, if an instructor demands excellence, students may bypass him and get checked by a more lenient instructor. The exacting instructor may then tend to lower his standards. On the other hand, if the instructor is too lenient, he may be chastised by his department chairman for laxness. Once again, this is one of the aspects of dental school teaching, i.e. interrelationships with patients as well as with students, that makes dental school teaching potentially more stressful than undergraduate college teaching.

Publish-or-Perish Philosophy and Research

The publish-or-perish philosophy is more relevant to college teaching. In dental schools, research and publications are not emphasized as much. Nevertheless, the more articles that are published and the more research that is done, the better the chances for tenure and promotion. The teacher-dentist-researcher is frustrated in those dental schools where research is de-emphasized.

Another possible source of frustration is the fact that some administrators and chairmen fail to reward for research and publications. This may be related to (1) jealousies, (2) lack of interest, (3) personality conflicts, or (4) the belief that research and publications should be secondary to actual teaching. In colleges and medical schools, there is usually a higher priority given to research and publications. Hopefully, more dental schools will realize that their image as a training school for turning out dental technicians will change if more emphasis is placed on basic and applied research and additions are made to the dental literature.

Summary

Dentist stress is multifactorial. It is related to the dentist's personality, the competition of schooling, the type of practice, and the dentist's social and family background. In Table 3-I, a questionnaire to assess dentist stress is presented. In this chapter, the sources of dentist stress have been covered. In Chapter 6, the management of dentist stress is discussed. In Chapter 4, the results of dentist stress are examined.

Table 3-I

THE DENTIST'S STRESS CHECK LIST*

It is said that half the battle is admitting to the obvious. How may items in the following check list can you claim?

Don't quibble; this is not a test. Remember, it's *your* health that is at stake.

__ Yes, I do bite my nails.
__ Yes, I brux, bite my cheeks, or clench my teeth.
__ Yes, I do have a tic, shake or tremble, hesitate in speech.
__ Yes, I have TMJ pain.
__ Yes, I do feel tense or keyed-up.
__ Yes, my heart pounds or races.
__ Yes, I do worry.
__ Yes, I do fidget, pace, or swear.
__ Yes, I do seethe or churn inside.
__ Yes, I do explode at times.
__ Yes, I do have a poor appetite.
__ Yes, I have difficulty falling asleep and staying asleep.
__ Yes, I feel everything is an effort and fatigue easily.
__ Yes, I am bored.

__ Yes, I do get headaches, shoulder pains, or low backaches.
__ Yes, I do get cold sores or rashes.
__ Yes, I do have ulcers or colitis.
__ Yes, I do have allergies.
__ Yes, I do have asthma.
__ Yes, I have had a coronary.
__ Yes, I have high blood pressure.
__ Yes, I do have diabetes.
__ Yes, I am overweight.

__ Yes, I'm a workaholic.
__ Yes, I do smoke.
__ Yes, I do drink more than one.
__ Yes, I do drink a great deal of coffee.

__ Yes, I do take sedatives or antianxiety drugs.

__ Yes, I have financial problems.
__ Yes, I'm having marital difficulties.
__ Yes, I have thoughts of ending my life.

__ No, I don't enjoy my practice.
__ No, I don't exercise regularly.
__ No, I don't get sufficient rest.
__ No, I don't have diversions.
__ No, I don't take periodic breaks.
__ No, I skip lunch.
__ No, my vacations don't restore me.

*The dentist should assess his stress in terms of the number of items he checks. While no minimum or maximum score is suggested, the object is to alert the dentist as to his present stress level.

REFERENCES

Chaney, C. A.: Stress and suicide. *Dent Surv, 53(6):*16, 1977.

Editorial: Dentists' debt and income rise — How do you compare? *PBP Update,* Sample Issue, 1977.

Editorial: The dentist's personal health problems — and some remedies. *Dent Surv, 52(7):*12, 1976.

Foley, W. J.: Stress from many sources affects your health and well being. *Dent Stud, 55(8):*34, 1977.

Gehrman, R.: In search of serenity. *Dent Manag, 17(12):*45, 1977.

Gold, C.: Stress and suicide. *Dent Surv, 53(6):*26, 1977.

Green, D.: The class of '76: How well are they winging it? *Dent Manag, 17(12):*22, 1977.

Howard, J. H., Cunningham, D. A., Rechnitzer, P. A., and Goode, R. C.: Stress in the job and career of a dentist. *JADA, 93:*630, 1976.

Igel, D. A.: Practicing under pressure. *Dent Surv, 52(2):*71, 1976.

Jackson, E. and Mealica, W. I., Jr.: Stress management and personal satisfaction in dental practice. *Dent Clin North Am, 21:*559, 1977.

Lamb, R.: Professional schools: Cram courses in tension and trauma. *New York Times Magazine,* 49, Nov. 20, 1977.

McClean, E. K. and Tarnopolsky, A.: Noise, discomfort and mental health. *Psychol Med, 7:*19, 1977.

McCollor, R. S.: A letter on dental stress. *Dent Econ, 67(3):*42, 1977.

Miller, N. E.: *Learning Effects on Somatic Manifestations of Stress.* Read before the Symposium on Stress and Behavioral Medicine. New York, Dec. 3-4, 1977.

Morse, D. R.: Overcoming "practice stress" via meditation and hypnosis. *Dent Surv, 53(7):*32, 1977a.

——: Variety, exercise, meditation can relieve practice stress. *Dent Stud, 56(3):*26, 1977b.

——: General practice, specialty or teaching. Which one's for you? *Dent Manag, 18(6):In Press,* 1978.

Protell, M. R., Krasner, J. D., and Fabrikant, B.: *Psychodynamics in Dental Practice.* Springfield, Ill., Thomas, 1975, pp. 3-22.

Redmond, P.: What your questionnaires told us about your health. *Dent Econ, 67(3):*28, 1977a.

——: What's behind the stress and strain of dentistry. *Dent Econ, 67(3):*39, 1977b.

Reyto, R.: Does the public ever appreciate us? *JADA 94:*435, 1977.

Riley, J. E.: Are dentists encouraging denturism? *Gen Dent, 25(6):*20, 1977.

Rosenbaum, V.: The explosive office triangle. *Dent Econ, 68(1):*80, 1978.

Schachter, S.: *The Psychology of Affiliation.* Stanford, Calif., Stanford U Pr, 1959.

Sharpe, F. L.: Dr. Black's school raises the roof over tuition. *Dent Manag, 56(1):*44, 1977.

Shaw, R. E.: Mercury is a hazard of your workplace. *Dent Stud, 55(8)*:26, 1977.

Sherlock, B. J. and Morris, R. T.: *Becoming a Dentist*. Springfield, Ill., Thomas, 1972.

Stressman, D.: My neighbor, the shrink. *Dent Econ, 67(4)*:74, 1977.

Sword, R. O.: The depression-prone personality: Almost "too good" to be true. *Dent Surv, 53(3)*:12, 1977.

——: Stress and suicide among dentists: Competitiveness and "being all things." *Dent Surv, 53(4)*:10, 1977.

Voss, L. and Shimoda, T.: Protect against free NO_2 in the operatory — for health's sake. *Dent Stud, 55(8)*:62, 1977.

Walters, E.: How to live with failure and stress. *Dent Manag, 16(10)*:20, 1976.

Wolfe, R. C.: Little things I learned from four malpractice suits. *Dent Manag, 18(2)*:21, 1978.

CHAPTER 4

THE RESULTS OF DENTIST STRESS

Consideration is given to (1) stress-related symptoms and diseases, such as cardiovascular diseases, malignancies, mental disorders, headaches, ulcers, diabetes, asthma, other hypersensitivity diseases, and miscellaneous diseases, such as tuberculosis and hyperthyroidism; and (2) stress-related disorders, such as alcoholism, drug addiction, smoking, obesity, partnership failures, divorce, and suicide.

INTRODUCTION

THE typical United States dentist is a paradox. He belongs to the profession that is rated by the public as being only second to medicine in prestige. He is an overachiever in high school, college, and dental school. Financially, he ranks close to the top of the country's income bracket. He uses the most advanced equipment, supplies, and techniques in the world, with the best supporting staff available. Typically, he is married, has a nice family, a beautiful home, at least two cars, and is well-thought-of in the community. He can choose his own working hours, take exotic vacations, and engage in all kinds of extracurricular activities. And yet, with all this, he is in a mess. A typical American dentist seems to be bent upon self-destruction. Dentists have been striving for parity with physicians for decades, and it seems that they have finally achieved it. Unfortunately, the parity is in stress-related diseases and disorders. These afflictions are now reviewed.

STRESS-RELATED SYMPTOMS AND DISEASES

Introduction

Stress is directly or indirectly related to a great number of diseases. There are certain stress manifestations that are common to many of these diseases. These include malaise, pain, fatigue, weakness, chills, sweating, high fever, insomnia, stomachaches, appetite loss, dizziness, and fainting. In addition to these non-specific responses, there are definitive changes for each particular disease.

While many people may be exposed to the same stress-inducing factors, some of them escape the development of stress-related diseases. It is not known why these people seem to be immune, but it is usually attributed to their higher stress-tolerance level. It is also not known why similar stressors result in different diseases for particular people. Probably all of the factors discussed in Chapter 1 under stressors and the individual makeup play a role in the development of stress-related diseases.

Certain of these factors seem to be more important in this respect. These include (1) the specific makeup of the individual, (2) the population and the virulence of the microbes or the potency of physical agents, (3) the particular environment, (4) the occurrence of major life-change events, and (5) the frequency of psychological stressors. The discussion that follows covers these five factors.

1. THE SPECIFIC MAKEUP OF THE INDIVIDUAL: In considering makeup, there are a number of major components that are thought to be significant in the determination of a given stress-related disease. These are (a) organ susceptibility, (b) inherited specificity of response patterns, (c) personality, (d) attitudes, (e) age period, (f) sex, (g) conditioning, and (h) occupation.

a. *Organ Susceptibility*. This concept, developed by H. G. Wolff (1953), states that people have inherent weaknesses in different organ systems. Thus, weakness of the gastrointestinal tract predisposes one to ulcers; a weakness of the respiratory system favors asthma development; and cardiovascular system weakness tends toward coronary artery disease.

b. *Inherited Specificity of Response Patterns*. The investigations of Lacey and Lacey (1958) have shown that particular individuals have highly stable and consistent autonomic nervous system response patterns. Some individuals repeatedly react to stress situations with a marked increase in heart rate; some respond with a dramatic rise in blood pressure; others show a major drop in skin resistance level (galvanic skin response); and still others respond with bronchial constriction. In Chapter 1, there was a discussion of sympathetic responders (sympathicotonics) and parasympathetic responders (vagotonics). Sympathicotonics with high blood pressure and rapid heart rate are prone to cardiovascular diseases; vagotonics with bronchial constriction tend toward asthma.

c. *Personality.* Some investigators have suggested that there is a specific personality type associated with each disorder. For example, descriptions are given for a "cancer personality" and an "ulcer personality." However, the associations are not clear-cut, except for Type A personality and coronary artery disease.

d. *Attitudes.* D. T. Graham and his associates (1962) have shown that the attitude of the individual influences the type of stress-related disease to which he is prone. Some examples are (1) an individual who feels deprived and wants to get even develops ulcers; (2) someone who is threatened with bodily harm and must be constantly prepared becomes hypertensive; (3) a person who feels neglected and wants to shut others out gets asthma; and (4) an individual who believes he is being injured or degraded and wants to get rid of the responsible agent comes down with colitis.

e. *Age Period.* In Chapter 1, the concept of normal life changes occurring in various age periods was discussed, e.g. Sheehy's *Passages.* Certain diseases may be more frequent for some people during potentially stressful periods, and such differences may relate to stress tolerance levels. Also, with advanced age, when immune responses are diminished, stress-related diseases become more prevalent, e.g. coronary disease, cancer, and adult-onset diabetes.

f. *Sex.* Prior to menopause, women are less prone than men to cardiovascular and infectious diseases (apparently related to estrogen). After menopause, women may be even more susceptible to coronary disease than men. Men appear to be genetically programmed to become bald (stressors add to the tendency). One recent study showed that "bald, fat men with hairy chests" had a greater chance of contracting heart disease (American Heart Association (1977).

g. *Conditioning.* As mentioned in Chapter 1, conditioning is important in the development of stress-related diseases. The level of conditioning varies with social status, motivation, financial means, and scientific background, e.g. knowing about the positive effects of exercise and nutrition. Conditioning has physical, mental, and nutritional components. (These three aspects are discussed under specific diseases.)

h. *Occupation.* Certain occupations by their nature are conducive to stress-related diseases. (These are discussed under cardiovascular diseases.)

2. VIRULENCE: The virulence of microbes and viruses and potency of other physical stressors greatly affects stress-related diseases. For example, many dentists are exposed to the tubercle bacillus but do not come down with tuberculosis. However, if a group of dentists came in contact with an overwhelming population of tubercle bacilli, then the chances of getting clinical tuberculosis would be very high for most of the group. Yet despite the exposure, some would remain free of disease (higher stress tolerance).

3. PARTICULAR ENVIRONMENT: Tuberculosis occurs more frequently in the poor who live in crowded cities. Rickets, which is causally related to lack of sunshine, is also more prevalent in such an environment. Stressors of city living include unsanitary conditions, cramped living quarters, and lack of sunshine.

4. OCCURRENCE OF MAJOR LIFE-CHANGE EVENTS: Petrich and Holmes (1977) and Rahe (1977) have developed a rating scale consisting of forty-three stressful life events. The major life-change events are numerically rated according to their potential for causing disease: death of a spouse = 100; divorce = 73 (Table 4-I). These events often antedate physical illnesses, such as coronary disease, ulcers, and severe infections. The more intense the life-change events and the higher the frequency of such events, the greater the chance for the subsequent development of a serious disease. On that stress scale, 200 or more stress

units in one year is considered to be potentially disruptive for most individuals. One other finding is that the major event may be good as well as bad and still create susceptibility to disease. For example, getting married rates 50 units. People vary in their ability to cope with these major stressors and also vary in their responses.

Table 4-I

REPRESENTATIVE RATINGS OF LIFE-STRESS EVENTS*

Rank	*Life Event*	*Mean Value*
1	Death of spouse	100
2	Divorce	73
4	Jail term	63
5	Death of close family member	63
7	Marriage	50
8	Fired at work	47
10	Retirement	45
13	Sex difficulties	39
15	Business adjustment	39
16	Change in financial state	38
17	Death of close friend	37
18	Change to different line of work	36
19	Change in number of arguments with spouse	35
21	Foreclosure of mortgage or loan	30
25	Outstanding personal achievement	28
28	Change in living conditions	25
30	Trouble with boss	23
32	Change in residence	20
40	Change in eating habits	15
41	Vacation	13

*Adapted from Petrich, J. and Holmes, T. H.: Life change and onset of illness. *Med Clin North Am, 61*:826, 1977.

5. Frequency of Psychological Stressors: Chronic day-to-day psychological stressors, such as anger, frustration, guilt, and anxiety, seem to be as important in the subsequent development of stress-related diseases as the sudden life-change events. As with major events, people's coping abilities vary, and the organs affected differ in individuals.

The occurrence of stress-related diseases appears to be linked to the outpouring of catecholamines and corticosteroids. In some diseases, the catecholamines are more important, e.g. coronary artery diseases. In other diseases, the action of the corticosteroids is predominant, e.g. gastric and duodenal ulcers. In contradistinction, there are diseases such as asthma, in which acetylcholine release (parasympathetic response) is predominant.

Next is an examination of the most prominent stress-related diseases, those of the cardiovascular system.

Cardiovascular Diseases

Introduction

Of all the stress-related diseases, the most significant are those of the cardiovascular system. Cardiovascular diseases include angina pectoris, atherosclerosis, hypertension, cardiac arrhythmias, coronary artery disease (coronary thrombosis or myocardial infarction), congestive heart failure, and cerebral stroke. Coronary artery diseases are the major cause of death in the United States. The National Heart, Lung and Blood Institute estimated that 1.3 million Americans presented with coronary disease in 1975. Of those, about 675,000 died, and 175,000 of them were premature deaths (under the age of sixty-five). A survey by the Bureau of Economic Research and Statistics of the ADA (1977) showed that myocardial infarctions and heart disease accounted for nearly 40 percent of all dentists' deaths (the major killer).

There are many risk factors for coronary heart disease, including (1) aging (disease increases with age); (2) sex (male incidence is higher than females); (3) elevated serum cholesterol and triglycerides; (4) hypertension; (5) heavy cigarette smoking, e.g. twenty or more cigarettes daily; (6) presence of diabetes mellitus; (7) parental history of coronary disease; (8) obesity; and (9) lack of physical exercise. Other factors that recently have been implicated are (1) high salt intake, (2) high carbohydrate intake, (3) the Type A coronary-prone personality, and (4) psychologic stressors. The last two factors listed are directly associated with stress and are now discussed.

Type A Personality

Friedman and Rosenman (1974) developed the concept of the Type A and Type B personalities and their relationship to stress-related diseases (primarily coronary disease). The Type B personality is seen as passive, restrained, not overly ambitious, and not prone to coronary disease. On the other hand, the Type A personality has characteristics, such as competitive achievement striving and feelings of time urgency, hostility, and aggressiveness, that are observed primarily in the presence of appropriate environmental circumstances. Type A persons are hard-drivers, i.e. compulsive, and they often set deadlines and quotas. They are impatient with delay, suppress fatigue and try to control their environment. When they are unsuccessful, they tend to become helpless. Type A's apparently are of the high risk category for coronary disease unless they learn to cope with their chronic day-to-day stressors. Many of these aspects of the Type A personality remind one of the description of behavioral patterns of dental students and dentists described in Chapter 3.*

Stress as a Causative Factor

There are many aspects of coronary artery disease that are influenced by stress. Although there are not always cause-and-effect relationships, and other factors are definitely of importance, stress certainly seems to be significant in the etiology of coronary disease. For instance, stress has caused increased blood cholesterol levels (Box 4-1).

Box 4-1: Cold Accountants and Cholesterol

Cold temperature and increased work-related stressors have

*One of the authors (D.M.) believes that he is a well-controlled Type A (only time will tell). The other (M.F.) considers himself to be a Type B who delights in aggravating Type A's.

been shown to raise blood cholesterol levels by as much as 100 mg% in a short time. This was dramatically shown with accountants during tax collection time (just prior to April 15 was the prime time). These levels tend to remain elevated during the entire period of "time pressure" (Eliot, 1977; Leff, 1975).

Psychological stressors employed in many animal and human experiments have been shown to increase blood pressure. Compared to psychological stressors, simple physical stressors were found not to be nearly as effective or consistent in terms of blood pressure elevation. Psychological stressors, such as frustration, conflict, crowding, and anxiety, caused the highest increases in blood pressure. When the psychological stressors were chronic, the blood pressure elevations remained at a higher state. Blood pressure did not return to normal after the cessation of the psychological stressors (Box 4-2).

It has been suggested that the chronic unresolved stress responses lead to an uncoupling between the alerted cardiovascular system and the inactive musculoskeletal system. (Fight-or-flight behavior cannot be invoked, as was done by our ancestors.) The state of readiness can be sustained for minutes, hours, days, weeks, or even longer. What probably happens is that there is a readjustment of the baroreceptors upward (the rheostat for blood pressure is set higher), which then results in chronic hypertension.

Box 4-2: Soaring Pressures

In human experiments, it has been shown that those same frustrated tax accountants (*see* Box 4-1) had sharp increases in their blood pressure during tax time. Students' levels go up before exams and so do soldiers' when they enter battle. In related experiments, Colb and Rose analyzed the activities and blood pressures of airport personnel. They found that air traffic controllers developed hypertension four times as frequently as second-class license controllers and did so seven years sooner in life. Hypertension occurred earlier in controllers working in towers with high-volume control as compared to those working towers with low-volume control (Glass, 1977; Leff, 1975).

Stressors have been shown to cause sustained elevation in blood catecholamine levels and studies have shown that catecholamines cause a sustained rise in blood pressure (Box 4-3).

Box 4-3: The Catastrophic Catecholamines

Catecholamines cause unique histopathologic changes in cardiac muscle (ruptured muscle fibers) that can result in sudden death. Catecholamines cause clumping of platelets, which are implicated in coronary thrombosis and also accelerate the rate of arterial damage, which can also be etiologically important in coronary thrombosis. Beta-blocking agents, e.g. Propranolol, cause a marked diminishing of the clinical manifestations of hypertension, angina pectoris, and ventricular extrasystoles. Beta-blockers interfere with sympathetic discharge. Their effectiveness suggests that the sympathetic catecholamines are important in the development of these three cardiac conditions (Editorial: Beta-blockers, 1976; Eliot, 1977; Glass, 1977).

In several retrospective and prospective studies, the relationship of recent life changes and myocardial infarction has been extensively studied (Petrich and Holmes, 1977; Rabkin and Struening, 1976; Rahe, 1977). Although the evidence is not overwhelming, it does appear that severe stress-inducing events such as the death of a loved one or loss of a job can greatly increase the chance of developing coronary disease or result in sudden death.

It also appears that many coronary victims have had bouts of anxiety and depression prior to their first signs of their disease. Therefore, chronic psychological stressors also appear to be of importance.

Summary

Considering that (1) many dentists are Type A individuals,

(2) dentists are subject to many chronic stressors in their daily lives, (3) dentists are in a relatively sedentary occupation, and (4) that divorce and marital problems (among other serious life events) may be in higher proportion for dentists than in the general population, it is not unusual that dentists suffer a high incidence of coronary disease. Methods of coping with the causes and effects of cardiovascular diseases are covered in Chapter 6.

Malignancies and Depression

Malignancies

The second leading killer of all diseases in the United States is cancer in one form or another. A survey of the Bureau of Economic Research and Statistics-ADA (1977) showed that cancer accounts for slightly more than 20 percent of all dentists' deaths and of the various types of cancer, dentists have a higher death rate from leukemia and pancreatic cancer than the rest of the population.

The etiology of malignancies is multifactorial and largely unknown in many instances. The relationship of malignancies to stress is less well understood than that of cardiovascular diseases to stress. Nevertheless, there is some evidence that cancer is often preceded by severe life changes and chronic psychologic stressors (Box 4-4).

Box 4-4: Cancer Prone

The great majority of studies of stress and cancer were clinical and based on personal experiences. A major theme reported was that anxiety, depression, hopelessness, and grief were significant precursors of the discovery of the malignancy. In one long-range prospective study at John Hopkins Medical School, Caroline Thomas found that physicians who developed cancer generally were "low-geared," had few outbursts of emotion, and had feelings of isolation from their parents that began in childhood.

In the other studies, often there was evidence of a major

loss, i.e. of a spouse or family member, immediately prior to the appearance of the cancer. An investigation by Lawrence Le Shan seemed to verify the conclusions about major life change prior to malignancies. He found that widowed persons had the highest cancer mortality rate and divorced individuals the next highest. In one study, people who had significantly higher depression scores on a personality test actually developed a significantly higher incidence of cancers than those individuals having a low depression index on the same test (Arehart-Treichel, 1977; Leff, 1975; Petrich and Holmes, 1977).

Depression

Richard Sword, a dentist-psychiatrist, recently discussed the attributes of the *depression-prone* personality (1977a). "It's a person who works hard, is ambitious, has a high sense of integrity, tells the truth, never gets mad, is very responsible and conscientious, pays bills on time (or at least tries to), is pleasant to everyone, smiles outwardly even when feeling like hell inside, has a strong sense of duty, and sets very high standards of performance for others but even more so for himself." That description sounds like the typical dental student-dentist, discussed in Chapter 3, who is subjected to many physical, psychological, and social stressors. There is some evidence that dentists do have a relatively high incidence of depression (Box 4-5 and Figure 4-1).

Box 4-5: The Depressed Dentist

In a recent survey by *Dental Economics* (Redmond, 1977a), 1,800 dentists responded to a questionnaire. Included was an analysis of depression. In the eastern United States (major cities), the highest incidence of depression was reported. Over 60 percent claimed some bouts of depression, with about 8 percent reporting being depressed often. In the *Dental Management* survey (1976) of the dental graduates of the University of Texas at Houston, more than one-half the class

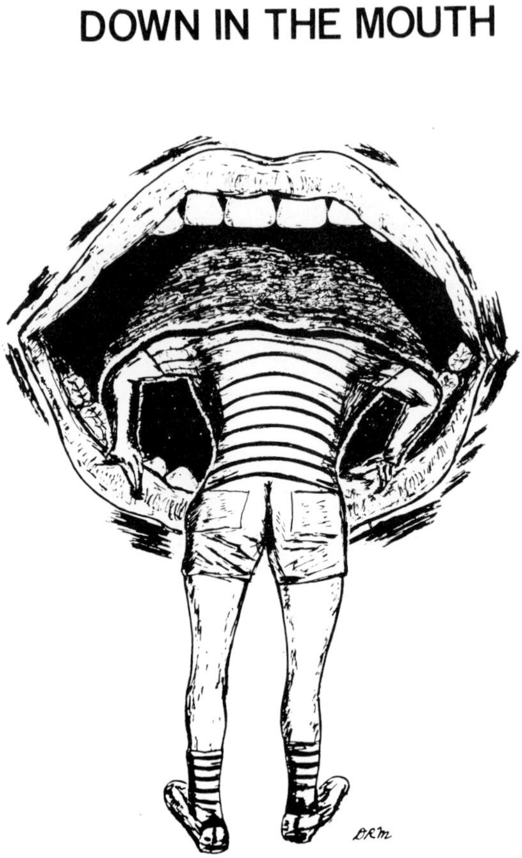

Figure 4-1. Down in the mouth. The depressed dentist may become so because he spends too much time working in the oral cavity (down in the mouth).

admitted that they had periods of depression (Green, 1977).

Depression may be of some importance in the etiology of malignancies (as just discussed), and it is a major factor in suicide. There is less evidence about the relationship to stress of other mental disorders, such as schizophrenia and paranoia. Yet, mental disorders in general and neurological diseases must be prevalent in dentistry, in light of a recent report that stated, "Nervous diseases were ranked as the third leading cause of death of dentists whereas it was ranked tenth as the cause of death in the general population (Foley, 1977).

Headaches, Shoulder Pains, and Backaches

Both tension and migraine headaches, as well as shoulder pains and backaches, are directly related to psychological stressors. Studies have shown that anxiety, anger, frustration, and worry act as precipitants in a substantial number of patients who have these conditions (Arehart-Treichel, 1977; Selye, 1976). Dental students and dentists are subject to these kinds of psychological stressors and many suffer from headaches, shoulder pains, and backaches (Norris, 1977).

Ulcers

In Selye's (1976) and Miller's (1977) studies, peptic ulcers occurred regularly in rats subjected to physical and psychological stressors. Brady (1958) showed that decision making could induce ulcers in monkeys and Seligman (1968) found that unpredictible pain was most effective in causing rat ulcers (Box 4-6).

Box 4-6: Executive Monkeys and Unpredictable Rats

An important investigation of psychosomatic disorders was conducted by Joseph Brady and his co-workers (1958). In Brady's experiment, "executive" and control monkeys were subjected to electric shock in which only the executive monkey could push a lever that would prevent both animals from receiving the shocks. Which monkey developed ulcers? The one with the responsibility. The studies also suggested that the ulcers occurred when the stressors were intermittent, rather than continuous, and when the occurrence of stress coincided with the natural periodicities of stomach secretions.

Moreover, unpredictable pain is even more likely to cause ulcers than predictable pain. This effect was discovered in an experiment by M. Seligman (1968), who compared the effects of unavoidable and unpredictable shocks in rats that did not receive a reliable warning signal with rats that did receive such a signal.

Taken together, these studies suggest that three major factors determine whether or not an aversive experience will lead to ulcers: (1) The more responsible an individual is for controlling the unpleasant events, the more he will be likely to experience stress and develop ulcers. (2) The less predictable the occurrence of the aversive event, the greater the anxiety and the higher the likelihood of developing ulcers. (3) The duration of the stressful experience and the timing of rest periods are crucial in determining whether or not ulcers will develop.

Gastric and duodenal ulcers occur in humans who suffer from such repeated psychological stressors as frustration, guilt, anger, and hate (Box 4-7).

Box 4-7: The Genesis of an Ulcer

The first clear evidence that ulcers can be produced in human beings by psychological stressors came from observations of a man whose esophagus had been so badly burned by scalding soup that the surgeon had to make a surgical opening directly into his stomach so that he could be fed. It then became possible to directly observe the formation of a painful ulcer in the lining of the stomach (Wolf and Wolff, 1943).

Duodenal ulcers have been shown to be preceded in many cases by major life-event changes, and there may be an "ulcer personality" (Box 4-8). There is also a correlation between O blood type and tendency toward ulcer development (Roberts, 1957).

Box 4-8: The Oral Ulcer

A prospective study by Herbert Weiner showed that there are certain primarily oral personality correlates with the development of ulcers. These include the desire to be fed, leaning on others, seeking close body contact with others, failure to express anger, and tendencies to be prim, tidy, mild, conscientious, inhibited, and punctual (Arehart-Treichel, 1977).

It seems that corticosteroid overproduction is apparently related to ulcers found in all three species, even though rat, monkey, and human ulcers may not be of the same kind. With humans, it is well known that latent ulcers can become activated and preexistant ulcers become worse when patients take corticosteroids.

Dentists daily face numerous psychological stressors and are often involved in decision making. Hence, it is not surprising that many dentists develop gastric and duodenal ulcers.

Diabetes Mellitus

Diabetes mellitus is one of the top five killers of all diseases in the United States. Although there is a strong genetic influence in the etiology, stress undoubtedly also plays a role. As mentioned in Chapter 1, both corticosteroids and catecholamines cause a rise in blood glucose, which, if sustained, could lead to diabetes in susceptible individuals. Both onset and exacerbation of adult-onset diabetes has been shown to be related to major life-change events. Diabetes is also a risk factor for coronary heart disease. Dentists are prone to this serious malady, although the reported incidence is not higher than that found in the general population.

Asthma and Other Hypersensitivity Diseases

Asthma is a serious, occasionally fatal, hypersensitivity disease that has a close relationship to stress. Unlike the cardiac diseases, asthma is precipitated by the release of acetylcholine and is relieved by catecholamines. Other hypersensitivity diseases that are also stress-related are chronic urticaria (hives), angioneurotic edema, hay fever, and vasomotor rhinitis (allergic cold). In all these conditions, both chronic psychologic stressors and major life-change events have been implicated as occurring prior to the onset of the diseases (Petrich and Holmes, 1977). About 15 percent of the population is reported to have allergies, and dentists are well represented with these conditions.

Miscellaneous Diseases

There are many other stress-related diseases and conditions, including tuberculosis, hyperthyroidism, rheumatoid arthritis, ulcerative colitis, neurodermatitis, premenstrual tensional syndrome, phlebitis, alopecia (loss of hair, baldness), graying of hair, dandruff, gout, arthritis, Cushing's disease, liver diseases, hypoglycemia, and infectious mononucleosis. The exact relationship with stress is tenuous, but some things are known. For instance, tuberculosis is exacerbated when corticosteroids are given exogenously. A similar result may also occur with stress. In a few studies, major life-change events preceded the onset of tuberculosis (Petrich and Holmes, 1977). During the stress response, thyroid hormones are released and metabolism increases, as discussed in Chapter 1. Development of hyperthyroidism could be precipitated as a result. Hyperthyroidism has been shown to occur at times following severe psychological or social stressors (Petrich and Holmes, 1977).

Recent studies have shown that most cases of rheumatoid arthritis occur in women (Arehart-Treichel, 1977). The disease seems to occur frequently in women who are unhappy in the traditional female sex role. The women are described as being frustrated, self-sacrificing, punctual, tidy, orderly, and perfectionists.

Ulcerative colitis development could be related to the irritant action on the colon of corticosteroids. Phlebitis may be related to the effect of catecholamines on platelet aggregation.* One study showed that uric acid is higher under certain stressful conditions; this could be a factor in the development of gout (Rahe et al., 1976). In Cushing's disease, there are high blood levels of corticosteroids. Dentists are as prone as anyone to develop one or more of these conditions (Box 4-8).

Box 4-8: The Aching, Hairless, Asthmatic Dentist

One of the authors (D.M.) developed an acute attack of

*Ex-President Nixon's development of thrombophlebitis may have been precipitated by the stressful events occurring in his life at that time (Leff, 1975).

asthma when he left the Army and again when he opened his first dental office. A few years later, he was under particularly strong stressors. Partly as a result, he developed vague neuralgia-like head pains and complete loss of facial hair (alopecia). Possibly by learning to cope in a more positive manner (discussed more fully in Appendix 1), the pains soon disappeared, the hair reappeared, and the asthma has not returned.

STRESS-RELATED DISORDERS

Introduction

DENTISTRY. DRUGS. DRINKING. DIVORCE. DEPRESSION. DEATH. What is the relationship of these six D's? The Bureau of Economic Research and Statistics of the ADA (1977) thinks there is little relationship. However, according to other surveys, dentistry and medicine are equal in the high incidence of drug addiction, alcoholism, divorce, depression, and suicide. Although there are little hard data for dentistry, there is more firm information for American medicine (Whieldon, 1977). Consider the following items: (1) The conservative estimates of the AMA state that one physician in twenty is impaired by drug abuse, alcoholism, or mental illness, and other estimates state that one in ten physicians are so involved. (2) Drug dependence is considered to be thirty to one hundred times more prevalent among physicians than among the general population. (3) Alcoholism affects almost 23,000 physicians (about 10% of the total) and almost one half of them mix drugs with drinks. (4) Depression is prevalent in medicine (in one eight-year study, almost half of the physicians hospitalized for alcohol, drug, or mental problems suffered from depressive neurosis). (5) Almost one half of physicians have unsatisfactory marriages, and many are divorced.

Drugs, Drinking, and Depression

Dentists are comparable to physicians in their (1) accessibility to drugs, (2) hard-driving personalities, and (3) self-reliance (rarely asking colleagues for help). There is some evidence that they are subject to the same disorders (Box 4-9).

Box 4-9: Drunk, Drugged, and Depressed

According to dentist-psychiatrist Richard Sword (1977a), dentists along with physicians "find it easier than others to start 'self-medicating' — and when they do, suicide can become a very real danger." Sword's findings are that drug dependence is just as high in dentistry as it is in medicine. The same is true for mixing drugs with alcohol and the incidence of depression. In the *Dental Economics* survey of 1,800 dentists in the United States, 5 percent reported that they go to a psychiatrist, and 32 percent reported being depressed (Redmond, 1977a).

Smoking and Obesity

As discussed in Chapter 2, both smoking and overeating can be used as means to cope with stressors. Millions of Americans smoke and overindulge in food, and dentists are well represented in their ranks. For example, the *Survey of Health Professionals: Smoking and Health, 1975* (National Clearinghouse, 1975) showed that 23 percent of dentists smoke, as compared to 21 percent of physicians.

Divorce and Business Breakup

Almost one half of all marriages in the United States end up in the divorce courts. While there are no reliable surveys with respect to dentistry, what information is available suggests that dentists are well represented in the divorce category. The stressors of practice and home life are partly responsible.

Similar factors may be involved in the failure of many dental partnerships and corporations. Another reason for the frequency of breakup may be related to the independence of dentists, a quality that is often accentuated in dental school training.

A Mixture

Stress has been shown to be related to drinking, eating, cardiovascular disease, psychological stressors, and divorce. An interesting mixture of these is discussed in Box 4-10.

Box 4-10: Paying the Price

A California cardiologist reported recently about extramarital sex and sudden death. According to Martin Krauthamer, it is not a question of retribution, but simply a matter of cause and effect. He states that cardiac arrest occurs more often with extramarital sex than when sexual involvement is with one's legal spouse. According to Krauthamer, there are usually the following compounding stressors: a strange partner, a heavy meal mixed with alcohol, strong guilt feelings, and a fear of detection. The prime candidate for a coronary attack is considered to be the forty-plus male who has a stressful occupation, eats poorly, and does not exercise, and, of course, is unfaithful (release from the *San Francisco Examiner* and reported in *Executive Fitness Newsletter,* 1977).

Suicide

Recent press releases and dental journal articles have stated that dentists have surpassed psychiatrists as being "Number 1 on the suicide parade." However, the evidence for this contention is debatable. Nevertheless, suicide appears to be a serious problem in dentistry. An editorial discussing this issue appeared in *Dental Management* (May, 1977) and is included in its entirety, since it presents an interesting review of dental suicide (Box 4-11).

Box 4-11: The Suicidal Dentist

Compared to the total U. S. population, are a disproportionate number of dentists destroying themselves each year?

The A.D.A. says no. Its recently issued study, based on the years 1960-65, concludes that "dentists had a composite death rate from all causes for each group that was less than that of the U. S. male population . . . And most importantly, deaths from suicide were not significantly different than that of the general white male population."

As for other publications which have come to different conclusions, the A.D.A. dismisses that as not based on "reliable research."

Way back in May of 1975, this magazine was the first dental publication to explore the whole question in a special issue devoted entirely to the dentist's physical and emotional health. We concluded back then that dentists were committing suicide at roughly *twice* the rate of the adult male population.

Our research source? The A.D.A.'s own figures, of course. A survey by its Bureau of Economic Research and Statistics, covering the years 1968-72, showed that 2.03 percent of the dentists who died during the period did so by their own hand (*JADA,* Jan., 1975). For the general population, according to figures developed by the Metropolitan Life Insurance Company, just 1.1 percent of all white, male deaths during the same period were suicides.

Metropolitan has long been known for its pioneering studies into mortality. Statisticians with the Met assured us that our comparisons were valid; our conclusions accurate.

All statistics on suicide are notoriously unreliable. Any man skilled enough to enter the dental profession is skilled enough to mask an unseemly exit from it. Yet, confirmation for these distressing figures comes from many sources.

• In a study of professional persons in Oregon, the suicide rate of attorneys, physicians, and dentists is three times that of white collar workers, with the dentists' rate the highest of all (*New England Journal of Medicine,* June, 1963).

• A study of health care professionals and technical workers in California shows dental suicides to be 83 per thousand, which was more than double the rate for the general population (*Archives of General Psychiatry,* Dec., 1973).

• In his landmark study, "Suicide and Attempted Suicide," Dr. Erwin Stengel, past president of the International Association for Suicide Prevention, concludes: "Medical and dental practitioners are among the professional groups with the highest suicide rates; they have more than double the rate of a comparable sample of the general population."

• A Study of New England dentists' mortality 1921-60 concludes that suicide "is the only cause of death with an excess (over the general population) approaching statistical significance over the entire study period" (Public Health Service Publication No. 999-RH-18).

We might understand the A.D.A. dismissing such reports as "not reliable research." More difficult to understand is why it has ignored the reports of its own research arm, the Bureau of Economic Research and Statistics, on dentists' suicide rates for 1968-72 and chosen instead to rely on the earlier period, 1960-65, for its latest announcement "refuting" the existence of a suicide problem in the dental profession.

That's enough of the numbers game, and the last time we shall play it at DENTAL MANAGEMENT. As long as the equivalent of one full dental graduating class continues to wipe itself out each year, we prefer to devote our time, our energies, and our editorial pages towards finding a solution. (Reprinted with permission of M. J. Goldberg, Editor *Dental Management,* and Harcourt Brace Jovanovich, Inc., New York, New York.)

Summary

There are disputes over the true incidence of stress-related diseases and disorders in dentistry. Nevertheless, stress is especially related to the development of coronary disease, depression, alcoholism, drug addiction, divorce, and suicide. There is no doubt that dentists develop these diseases and disorders.

Therefore, it is important that dentists are aware of them and learn means of coping with these afflictions. In Chapter 6, the management of stress-related dentists' diseases and disorders is covered. In the next chapter, the management of patient stress and stress-related oral diseases is considered.

REFERENCES

American Heart Association: *Risko: A Way to Alert You to the Risks of Heart Attack.* Columbus, Ohio Affiliate, 1977.

Arehart-Treichel, J.: Can your personality kill you? *New York Magazine, 10:*62, Nov. 28, 1977.

Benson, H.: Systemic hypertension and the relaxation response. *N Engl J Med, 296:*1152, 1977.

Brady, J. V.: Ulcers in "executive monkeys." *Sci Am, 199(4):*95, 1958.

Bureau of Economic Research and Statistics-ADA: The occupation of dentistry: Its relation to illness and death. *JADA, 95:*606, 1977.

Cassem, N. H. and Hackett, T. P.: Psychological aspects of myocardial infarction. *Med Clin North Am, 61:*711, 1977.

Cutright, D. E., Carpenter, W. A., Tsaknis, P. G., and Lyon, T. C.: Survey of blood pressure of 856 dentists. *JADA, 94:*918, 1977.

deChamplain, J. and Cousineau, D.: Lack of correlations between age and circulating catecholamines in hypertensive patients. *N Engl J Med, 297:*672, 1977.

Editorial: Beta-blockers in anxiety and stress. *Br Med J, 2:*415, Feb. 21, 1976.

Editorial: The heart of the type A debate. *Med World News, 16:*103, Feb. 24, 1975.

Editorial: The penalty of sin. *Exec Fitness Newsletter,* Sample Issue 1, 1977.

Editorial: Two studies list major cause of dentists' deaths. *PBP Updäte,* Sample Issue, 1977.

Eliot, R. S.: Stress and cardiovascular disease. *Eur J Cardiol, 5(2):*97, 1977.

Engel, G.: Emotional stress and sudden death. *Psychol Today, 10(11):*114, 1977.

Foley, W. J.: Stress from many sources affects your health and well being. *Dent Stud, 55(8):*34, 1977.

Friedman, M. and Rosenman, R. H.: *Type A Behavior and Your Heart.* New York, Knopf, 1974.

Friedman, R. and Iwai, J.: Genetic predisposition and stress-induced hypertension. *Science, 193:*161, 1976.

____ : Hypertension and the nature of stress. *Science, 198:*80, 1977.

Glass, D. C.: Stress, behavior patterns and coronary disease. *Am Sci, 65:*177, 1977.

Goldberg, M. J.: The numbers game. *Dent Manag, 17(5):*10, 1977.

Graham, D. T., Lundy, R. M., Benjamin, L. S., and Kabler, F. K.: Some specific attitudes in initial interviews with patients having different "psychosomatic" diseases. *Psychosom Med, 24:*257, 1962.

Green, D.: The class of '76: How well are they winging it! *Dent Manag, 17(12):*22, 1977.

Hurst, M. W., Jenkins, C. D., and Rose, R. M.: The relation of psychological stress to onset of medical illness. *Ann Rev Med, 27:*301, 1976.

Jenkins, C. D.: Recent evidence supporting psychologic and social risk factors for coronary disease. *N Engl J Med, 294:*987, 1976.

Kagan, A.: A stressless definition of "stress" and some speculations on its relationship to cardiovascular disease. *Acta Cardiol T (Brux), 30:*331, 1975.

Lacey, J. I. and Lacey, B. C.: Verification and extension of the principle of autonomic response stereotype. *Am J Psychol, 71:*50, 1958.

Lamb, R.: Professional schools: Cram courses in tension and trauma. *New York Times Magazine,* 49, Nov. 20, 1977.

Leff, D. N.: Stress-triggered organic disease in this year of economic anxiety. *Med World News, 16:*74, Mar. 24, 1975.

Lynch, J. J., Paskewitz, D. A., Gimbel, K. S., and Thomas, S. A.: Psychological aspects of cardiac arrhythmia. *Am Heart J, 93:*645, 1977.

Mansky, M.: Suicide. *Dent Manag, 17(5):*83, 1977.

Marx, J. L.: Stress: Role in hypertension debated. *Science, 198:*905, 1977.

Miller, N. E.: *Learning Effects on Somatic Manifestations of Stress.* Read before the Symposium on Stress and Behavioral Medicine. New York, Dec. 3-4, 1977a.

Miller, N. E. and Dworkin, B. R.: Effects of learning on visceral functions — Biofeedback. *N Engl J Med, 296:*1274, 1977b.

National Clearinghouse for Smoking and Health and the National Cancer Institute: *Survey of Health Professionals: Smoking and Health, 1975,* U.S. Gov't Publ., Wash, D.C.

Norris, C.: Is your back biting back? *Dent Manag, 17(11):*57, 1977a.

——— : Suicide. *Dent Manag, 17(5):*84, 1977b.

Petrich, J. and Holmes, T. H.: Life change and onset of disease. *Med Clin North Am, 61:*825, 1977.

Rabkin, J. G. and Struening, E. L.: Life events, stress and illness. *Science, 194:*1013, 1976.

Rahe, R. H.: *Life Stress Events and Illness.* Read before the Symposium on Stress and Behavioral Medicine. New York, Dec. 3-4, 1977.

Rahe, R. H., Ryman, D. H., and Biersner, R. J.: Serum uric acid, cholesterol, and psychological moods throughout stressful naval training. *Aviat Space Environ Med, 47:*883, 1976.

Reading, A.: Illness and disease. *Med Clin North Am, 61:*703, 1977.

Redmond, P.: What your questionnaires told us about your health. *Dent Econ, 67(3):*28, 1977a.

____ : What's behind the stress and strain of dentistry. *Dent Econ, 67(3):*39, 1977b.

Rees, W. L.: Stress, distress and disease. *Br J Psychiatry, 128:*3, 1976.

Roberts, J. A. and Fraser, C.: Blood groups and susceptibility to disease. *Br J Prev Soc Med, 11:*107, 1957.

Rose, K. D. and Rosow, I.: Physicians who kill themselves. *Arch Gen Psychiatry, 29:*800, 1973.

Seligman, M.: Chronic fear produced by unpredictable electric shock. *J Comp Physiol Psychol, 66:*402, 1968.

Selye, H.: *The Stress of Life,* 2nd ed. New York, McGraw, 1976.

Sniderman, M.: Attitudes toward health professions. *Pa Dent J, 43(11):*5, 1976.

Stumpf, W. E., Sar, M., and Aumüller, G.: The heart: A target organ for estradiol. *Science, 196:*319, 1977.

Sword, R. O.: The depression-prone personality: Almost "too good" to be true. *Dent Surv, 53(3):*12, 1977a.

____ : Stress and suicide among dentists: Competitiveness and "being all things." *Dent Surv, 53(4):*10, 1977b.

Ulene, A.: *Feeling Fine.* Los Angeles, J. P. Tarcher, 1977.

Walters, E.: How to live with failure and stress. *Dent Manag, 16(10):*20, 1976.

Whieldon, D.: Drinkers, addicts, depressives: What happens when they're doctors? *Pract Psychol Physicians, 4(11):*13, 1977.

Wolf, S. and Wolff, H. G.: Evidence of the genesis of peptic ulcer in man. In Tomkins, S. S. (Ed.): *Contemporary Psychopathology.* Cambridge, Mass., Harvard U Pr, 1943.

Wolff, H. G.: *Stress and Disease.* Springfield, Ill., Thomas, 1953.

CHAPTER 5

OVERCOMING PATIENT STRESS

Methods of overcoming patient fear and the negative office atmosphere are considered. The following are covered: (1) education; (2) the pleasant office atmosphere; (3) the drugless approaches, including "chairside manner," patient control, behavior modification, progressive relaxation, autogenic training, hypnosis, meditation, biofeedback, audioanalgesia and massage; and (4) the drug methods, including sedatives, antianxiety agents, effective local anesthesia, conscious sedation, and general anesthesia. Methods of treating stress-related oral diseases are discussed, including the use of behavior modification, hypnosis, meditation, biofeedback, antianxiety agents, exercise, electrical stimulation, and acupuncture.

OVERCOMING FEAR AND OFFICE-RELATED PROBLEMS

Introduction*

Situation 1

THE fingernails dig into the armrests, and trickles of sweat run down the sleeves. The whole body stiffens as the needle ominously advances towards its oral destination. As the needle pierces, your heart is pounding and you scream inwardly, praying that it will take over quickly. Soon the pain dissipates as the numbness supervenes. Now your eyes scan and your ears listen, awaiting the next happening: the drilling. And it begins — the whirling bur, the screeching whine. As the bur sinks into the tooth, you sink into the chair. It doesn't hurt, but you're clenching and anticipating, filled with mixed feelings. ("I can't stand the numbness, but I hope it's numb enough.")

*From D. R. Morse: The Practice Building Spell, *Dental Survey, 54(3)*:20, 1978. Courtesy of Dental Survey Publications and Harcourt Brace Jovanovich, Inc., New York, New York.

From the start the saliva flows, but the saliva ejector is doing its job and you're drying up. Now the little monster is attacking your tongue and the floor of your mouth. It's almost as if there were two counteracting forces — the drill pushing you down, the saliva ejector pulling you up.

You count the seconds; the drill lifts up from the tooth; you sigh with relief. An explorer checks the preparation; the drill is reactivated. This cycle continues for awhile. Just when you've "had it," the drill is put to rest. Next, a clamp is placed around the tooth and under the gum. Then it is tightened. You feel as if the tooth and gum is being crushed, but the unpleasant sensation soon goes away. Then the filling begins. In goes a portion of silver, followed by pushing and packing. ("If he's filling my tooth, why do I feel it in my brain?")

Finally, the condensation is complete, the clamp is removed, and the carving begins. That part is best. ("But why does he have to carve his initials?") As the saliva ejector is removed, you wipe your mouth, thank the dentist and assistant, and bolt out of the chair.

You reluctantly stop off at the desk, pay the bill, and discuss the next appointment. "Mr. Brown, can you come in this Tuesday at the same time?" "I'm sorry, Miss Jones, I'll be out of town for the next two weeks (probably a lie); I'll call for my next appointment." As you leave, you have to admit that modern dentistry is painless, but you still must postpone the appointment. ("After all, how can going to the dentist be enjoyable!")

Situation 2

The eyelids flutter, and as they close you feel yourself slowly sinking into the contoured chair. All of your body's muscles uncoil, and soon you are surrounded by silence. Yet, within yourself, the feelings are intense.

It begins with a slight tingling of the toes. This is soon followed by minipulsations of the fingertips. These pleasant vibrations then spread throughout the body. The heart beats slower, and the mouth gets drier. Your body feels suspended in space, relieved of weight, and relieved of tension. The mind then begins to unfold its images, and the trip begins.

"Open please!" You hear his voice and you open your mouth, but in your mind, a scene appears. It starts with a yellow haze that gradually dissipates. As the view unfolds, a typical beach scenario is evident. (The dentist turns on the operating light.) The sunlight is intense, the sea is calm, the sand glistens, and *you* are there.

(The dentist injects the local anesthetic.) You feel a slight pinch but you don't mind it, because you're somewhere else. You don't question how you got there or why you chose that place. You just accept the reality of the moment and become part of it.

After a while your mouth feels numb, but so do your arms and legs. In fact, your whole body feels numb, light, and suspended. (The dentist adjusts the light and begins to drill.) You feel the warmth of the light and hear the sound of the drill and you think, "The sun is really intense today; that water looks inviting; I think I'll take a swim." The waves bounce gently onto the shore, and you let the lukewarm water caress your body.

Still, there is a dichotomy — part of you is back in the dental office, sitting in the chair, having a tooth fixed — part of you is squinting from the sun while sitting in nature's water bed. But you don't care, and you continue the trip.

(The dentist inserts the band and begins to condense the amalgam.) You feel some pressure now and it sends a slight chill down your spine. Then the day changes and the water is colder. You swim out into the ocean and approach an isolated island. You hop onto dry land, flop onto the sand, and the warmth pervades your body.

(The dentist removes the band and carves the filling.) There is no pressure now and no cold sensation, only the tickle from the carving. In your mind's eye, you look around and see a field of flowers, daisies in bloom. You touch them and they engulf you, enrapture you. The fragrance is magnificent. You smell it in that distant field and it too becomes part of the dental office.

"When you are ready, you can rinse out your mouth." You

hear his voice. You feel such inner calm, but you know it is time, and time takes precedence. So you begin to move and the mist returns. You stretch, and darkness supervenes. You sigh, open your eyes, and rinse out your mouth.

You slowly get out of the chair and practically float to the front desk, feeling so relaxed. You pay the bill and willingly confirm next week's appointment. As you leave, you think about that enjoyable trip and look forward to another one soon.

* * * * *

Although situations 1 and 2 are hypothetical, they illustrate the varying experiences patients can have in the dental situa-

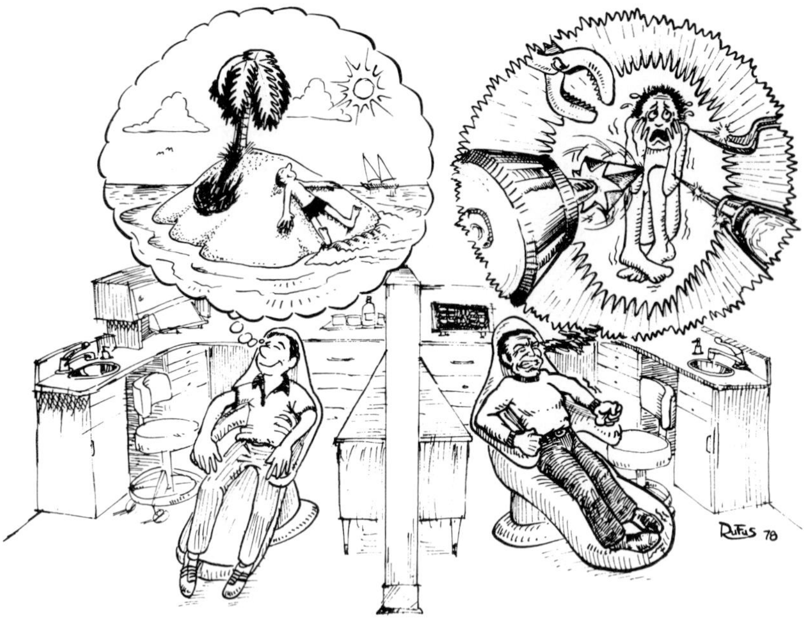

B **A**

Figure 5-1. Two dental patient situations: (*A*) Situation 1, an apprehensive patient, anticipating the worst. (*B*) Meditating patient, taking a pleasant mental trip, Situation 2.

tion (Fig. 5-1). The different methods that promote favorable patient reactions, such as the self-hypnosis in situation 2, are now considered. Recommendations are made with respect to the dentists' image, the dental media, and the use of dental terms. The reader should bear in mind that what follows is based on a combination of practical experience, art, and science.

Education

As indicated in Chapter 2, fear is a primary deterrent to dental treatment, and a major source of this fear is negative dental experiences. The past surely cannot be changed, but the public should be made aware of the various means of pain and anxiety control that are currently available.

Although modern dentistry is approaching the twenty-first century, the dentists' image is mired in the late nineteenth century when dentistry was an offshoot of barbering and smithery, e.g. barbers and silversmiths practiced dentistry without having any medical training. The reason for the negative image is fourfold. The first is that it is generally the bad news and, especially, bad experiences that make the headlines. People love to relate horror stories and tales of woe, and the stories become worse in the retelling. Undoubtedly, there are some dentists who practice with antiquated equipment and methods, but patients' pleasant or neutral experiences are rarely repeated. In fact, most patients do not go into shock at the sight of a needle or from hearing the sound of a drill. In addition, most dentists perform high-quality work in a pleasant, relaxed office atmosphere.

The second reason for the negative image has to do with dentistry's sister profession, medicine, which often exacerbates this image. Consider this introductory statement in an editorial in the *Journal of the American Medical Association* (Vaisrub, 1975): "Visions of needles, drills, forceps and probes greatly detract from the attractions of the dentist's chair for its prospective occupants." Medical practitioners should be educated about the advances in dentistry; they often are as fearful as anyone else, and many of their mouths are living testimonies to that fact.

The third reason has to do with the media. Whenever a dentist is portrayed in the newspapers, magazines, TV, novels, or artwork, it is always in a debasing or humorous* manner. He is the man who inflicts pain; a meek sorrowful soul, often shown with glasses, partially bald, and stooped. He is even portrayed as evil. Consider the uncanny combination of a Nazi dentist as the villain in William Goldman's *Marathon Man* (1974).

The fourth reason for the negative image is self-induced. Dentists should be proud of their profession. They work in a small, circumscribed area, use fine, delicate instruments, and often must use a mirror to operate by indirect vision. The treatments are highly sophisticated. No other health professional, with the possible exception of the neurosurgeon, works so delicately. (For instance, consider the skill required for instrumentation and obturation of the fine, curved root canals of an upper molar.) Dentists work on a conscious, often fearful, patient whose slightest movement can contravene good results. And with all of this, dentists generally get good results. The fact is that dentistry is demanding and dentists perform an important service. Dentists should be proud of their profession, and they should receive positive recognition for their achievements. The time of the reticent dentist is past.

How can the negative image be changed? Communication may be the answer. Dentists should write articles for the lay press. They should appear on radio and TV programs as invited professionals with an important message. They should address local clubs and organizations. Dentists can and should influence their acquaintances and neighbors via friendly persuasion. They should talk with their medical colleagues. The

*The publication of many humorous cartoons and anecdotes may be related to three factors: (1) Humor is a stress-release mechanism, and the dental situation is stress producing. (2) Humor is a means for the involved artists and writers to overcome their fears about dental treatments. (3) Humor is a way for the individuals to "get even" with their dentists for inflicting pain.

ADA should take a bigger role in mass media advertising. In dental offices, the entire staff should be trained to make positive presentations. The use of patient education, pamphlets, and audiovisual machines can be valuable if reinforced by encouraging remarks from the staff.

Office Atmosphere

In regard to office atmosphere, the physical layout, the dentist, and his staff are now discussed.

The Physical Layout

Positive presentation can only be effective if the atmosphere is conducive to relaxation. There is no right way to decorate an office. Each month for several years, *Dental Survey* magazine has featured a "beautiful" dental office. The layouts are all different, and yet they all have some common features. First and foremost, the office should not have a cold, stark, hospital-like appearance. The colors should be warm: Referring back to Chapter 2, blue typifies security and comfort; yellow generates joy and happiness.

When talking to patients, it is suggested that dentists should use the term *reception room*. This phrase implies bringing someone into a pleasant place, such as the living room of one's home. *Waiting room* means the patients are expected to wait, and most people do not like to wait. The furniture in the reception room should be inviting. The chairs should appear comfortable. There should be colorful drapes, warm carpeting, plants, and decorative, pleasant lighting. The magazines should be current (dated periodicals seem to go hand in hand with antiquated dentistry).

Some dentists serve wine or other mild alcoholic beverages in the reception room to relax their patients, but this could be a problem with alcoholics. It could also interfere with the patient's driving home after the appointment. Serving coffee or tea is not necessary, but many patients appreciate it as a sign of hospitality and caring.

Since dentists are concerned with health, smoking should be discouraged. Therefore, ashtrays should not be present in the reception room, and the staff members should not smoke (at least not in the presence of patients). If a patient must smoke to relieve anxiety, the dental staff should not add to his burden by insisting he not smoke. Possibly, the receptionist could invite the patient to smoke in an area allocated outside the office (perhaps in the rest room).

The room temperature should be comfortable. If possible, there should be an interesting view visible from the reception room window. If that is not feasible because of location, pictures of relaxing scenes could decorate the walls. There should not be signs screaming out at the patients, such as "Payment is expected per visit," or "There will be a charge for broken appointments." If these rules are office policy, they can be stated in a discreet manner either when discussing the treatment plan or later.

In a dental office, most people accept semiclassical music played quietly in the background; some might prefer other music at times, such as rock, folk, or classical music, but usually not in a dentist's office.

It is suggested that the treatment rooms not be called *operatories*. This term implies that major operations are to be performed. Soft, contoured chairs, recessed equipment, carpeted floors, and pleasant wall and window decorations can add to the relaxing atmosphere in the treatment rooms. Other means of allaying anxiety are (1) use of the vibration-free, ultra-high-speed handpiece (anyone who has had a tooth prepared with a slow-speed handpiece, even with good anesthesia, remembers the terrible heat and vibration generated); (2) having the dentist wash his hands in the presence of the patient (to allay fear about transmission of infection); (3) use of disposable supplies (again to show concern about sterility); (4) use of a red mouthwash to decrease the apprehension that might arise from seeing blood in the cuspidor; and (5) use of pleasant, scented sprays or freshly cut flowers to mask the treatment room odors.

The Staff

Most dentists and their aides have turned to the use of either soft, pastel colors, tan, or plaid for their uniforms to offset the fear of "the man in white." It is also imperative that the dentist and his staff members be impeccably groomed. They must look and smell clean. Attention to these matters of personal appearance helps promote an atmosphere of caring and relaxation.

The first contact the patient makes with the dental office is usually via the telephone. It is essential that the receptionist speak to the patient in a pleasant, positive, and sympathetic way.

Studies have shown that the most appropriate time and place to begin to reduce patient anxiety is in the reception room before treatment has begun (Lamb and Plant, 1972). The new patient should be greeted by the receptionist and dentist in an open, warm, friendly manner. If delays are necessary, a courteous, honest explanation should be given. Financial arrangements should be discussed privately by the receptionist (or by the dentist if special problems arise) after the dentist has taken care of the patient's major complaint.

The Dentist

The dentist should also project a warm, friendly image to his patients. Most authorities believe that anxiety is reduced if case presentations are done in the consultation rather than in a treatment room (Bloomfield, 1962). The consultation room should not be called the *private office* because that term implies it is reserved for the doctor. *Consultation* infers mutual consideration and is a preferred term.

As mentioned previously, the desk can be both a physical and mental barrier to rapport. Some practitioners, even if they have a desk, sit side by side with the patient when they discuss the case (Box 5-1).

Box 5-1: The "X-Rayted" Skull

With respect to case presentations, Loren Borland (1962) has found that some patients become distressed at the viewing of x-rays. For these patients, x-rays are portions of the skull, and a skull symbolizes death. The same rationale may be operating for some patients who are reluctant to view study models. Borland's comments are apropos. "On the whole, patients do not wish to think about the unpleasant aspects of what is wrong with them. If they accept the dentist as a person and as an adequately trained professional man whom they can trust, they will unquestioningly accept his suggestions and evaluations and be much less apprehensive as a result."

It is incumbent upon all professionals to periodically return to school for refresher courses and keep up with the literature of their discipline. Adhering to this concept should enhance the dentist's image with his patient. A patient who has confidence in his doctor's ability is under less stress.

The mannerisms and voice of the dentist, along with his staff, should also be conducive to relaxation. Obviously, yelling at patients and staff members should never be done. If some disciplinary action is necessary, it should take place in private. Studies have shown that either loud or hesitant and halting speech induces anxiety and negative feelings (Baseheart, 1975).

Dentists should use simple, positive words when speaking to patients. Dentists should avoid technical language and eliminate anxiety-producing words or phrases, such as *needle, hot, drill, filling, hate, pain, nerve, plates, cavities, dead tooth,* and *mouth rehabilitation.* Positive or neutral substitutes for the preceding words or phrases are *dislike, discomfort, injection* or *syringe, handpiece, restoration, mouth restoration, decay, dentures, pulpless* or *nonvital tooth,* and *pulp* (Box 5-2).

Box 5-2: The Negative Needle

In a study at Temple University, the authors found that the negative word *needle* induced stressful physiological responses to subjects who were meditating and had previously shown physiologic signs of deep relaxation. Physiological measures used were pulse rate, respiratory rate, and skin resistance levels and fluctuations. When questioned later, most of the subjects stated that they felt highly anxious when they heard the word *needle* (Morse et al., 1978).

Not only are the kinds of words used important, but also the tone of the voice can induce either fear or relaxation, depending upon the quality and pitch. A quiet, soothing voice can help a patient overcome his anxieties.

Body language can be effective in increasing or decreasing anxiety. A dentist leaning back on his chair might be conveying a more negative attitude to a patient than if the dentist was leaning forward. Eye contact is very important to generate trust and reduce apprehension (Box 5-3).

Box 5-3: The Friendly Eye

Studies have shown that the greater the friendliness between two people, the greater the eye contact. "Warm" people display much more eye contact toward others than do "cold" people; and subjects reported higher ratings of "liking" with increased periods of eye contact (Baseheart, 1975).

The dentist should look at his patients when he speaks and really listen to them when they speak. The dentist should not think that a patient is stupid if he asks the dentist to repeat something or if he keeps repeating the same phrase himself. Sometimes the point is too technical, and the patient needs a simpler explanation; other times he wants reassurance; or he may want additional reasons to justify the time and expense involved. Furthermore, the patient may be under stress and experiencing tunnel vision, in which the perception of stimuli is reduced. The patient may also want the dentist to help him overcome his anxieties and often simply wants the dentist to listen to his problems. There is much to the old maxim, "A shared grief lessens, a shared joy increases."

Finally, if a patient can no longer control his emotions, he should be encouraged to cry. Crying is an effective stress-release mechanism that should not be inhibited.

The Drugless Approaches

Introduction

There are various nondrug methods that can aid in the reduction of patient stress. These may vary from the use of a calm, reassuring chairside manner to the use of elaborate biofeedback equipment. Whatever the method used, the desired end result is to have a relaxed patient receiving optimal dental care.

The Chairside Manner

The bedside manner went out with the house visits of the old family doctor. But a gentle chairside manner by the dentist in dealing with his patients can help in reviving this approach. The dental assistant can be helpful in this respect by helping the patient remove hats, wraps, purses, or packages. She should solicitously assist the patient into the chair. A gentle, reassuring touch on the shoulder by the assistant or doctor can help assuage the patient's fears. But it must be remembered that some patients become offended by being touched, so this should be kept to a minimum and used only for the most apprehensive patients.

It is also important that the concept of personal space be kept in mind. The dentist should not hover over patients. It is even a good idea for the dentist (as well as for the patient's benefit) to occasionally interrupt the clinical procedure to get up, stretch, and leave the room; a "breather" is always beneficial.

With children, there are other ways to offset anxiety. Some dentists successfully use materials such as games and toys in the reception room, TV in the treatment room, and magician's tricks in both places. Murray Simon (1976) has given a fascinating description of the magic techniques he uses to overcome fear and gain confidence. One method that is used with children is the "tell, show, do" game. With this technique, there is no actual treatment attempted during the first visit; it is a get-acquainted session; the child learns about the office and the equipment, and there are no hidden surprises. Studies have shown that even when children have extractions, proper preparation time greatly reduces the anxiety levels (Baldwin, 1966). Thus, it can be said that a gentle approach is effective with people of all ages.

Patient Control

One of the fears some patients have is loss of control. A patient may feel helpless or trapped, unable to escape the situation. Some methods that dentists have used to overcome this fear are the following: (1) Allow the patient to hold a hand mirror in one hand to observe what is happening (reassuring to some; others might find it disturbing). (2) Install a push button that the patient can press to stop the drilling when it gets uncomfortable (Box 5-4). (3) Let the patient raise his hand when he wants the dentist to stop. (4) Give the patient a degree of control to deepen or lighten their states with the use of audioanalgesia and nitrous oxide-oxygen analgesia set ups.

Box 5-4: The Obedient Drill

Loren Borland (1962) installed a patient-controlled push button on his dental unit. The patients were informed that if the drilling became bothersome, merely pushing the button would cause the drill to stop. It was found that the patients generally only depressed the button within the first few minutes of drilling. Once they were reassured that they did have control, they no longer used it.

Patients may also fear that they will have no control after they leave the office. Hence, it is imperative that explicit instructions relative to drugs and irrigation, etc., are given and the patient is told that he can contact the doctor in case of any subsequent dental problem.

Behavior Modification

Behavior modification is the alteration of undesirable behaviors to more acceptable ways of functioning. The methods are derived from psychological and learning theories. Techniques applicable to management of dental fears are as follows: (1) positive and negative reinforcement (contingency management); (2) modeling; (3) role playing (behavioral rehearsal); (4) systemic desensitization (reciprocal inhibition); and (5) forced exposure (flooding).

1. Contingency Management: Contingency management involves the giving (positive) or taking (negative) of reinforcers to increase the probability of a designated behavior. Giving the child a toy at the completion of the visit as a reward for being a good patient is a positive reinforcer. The child should be given a gift only if the desired behavior is manifested. In some offices, children are given toys regardless of how they behave. Indiscriminate reinforcement is not an appropriate way to reward a child in the hope that he will become a better patient. Yet, there is some evidence that giving a child a reward, e.g. a "magic penny," before the treatment may be more meaningful and helpful than giving a gift at the completion of the treatment (Box 5-5). For adults as well as for children, a kind word, a handshake, and a smile are effective positive reinforcers.

Box 5-5: The Transparent Bribe

In a study by Lund and Kegeles, the use of positive reinforcers was examined. The goal was to get children to use a special mouthwash each day. There were three groups: Group A received a reward for cooperating, e.g. a transistor radio; group B was involved in regular discussions about the importance of dental care; and group C was just asked to use the mouthwash. It was found that group B did the worst, probably showing that even young children don't like to talk about dentistry. Group A, i.e. those who were rewarded, did the best, but only half of them continued to use the mouthwash for the entire duration of the experiment (Hassett, 1978).

Negative reinforcement is less frequently used. It involves the use of punishment to eliminate or reduce the unwanted behavior. What may be happening is that the unwanted behavior is blocked temporarily, so that the probability of a more desirable behavior is increased. This may then be positively reinforced for subsequent performance. Negative reinforcement may be expressed by words, physical action, a disapproving nod, or a frown. The use of the towel technique (*see* Chap. 2) to control resisting children, may be considered a poor example of negative reinforcement. Most authorities recognize that the towel technique is less than an effective means to reduce fear (Schwartz, 1975). Subtle use of words and facial expressions may be more effective with both children and adults both in dealing with resistance and with lessening the fear reaction.

2. Modeling: Modeling is a means to effect behavioral change by having an individual watch a model of behavior. Modeling can be effectively used in the dental office to overcome the dental fears of children and apprehensive adults. The usual arrangement is to have the child watch his mother, sibling, or friend undergoing dental treatment. If the model is a good dental patient and does not display any evidence of pain or anxiety, then the procedure may work. Audiovisual films can also be used effectively to demonstrate pain and anxiety-free dentistry (Box 5-6). Modeling can be employed in the office or may be used with larger groups in a school or clinic.

Box 5-6: The Film Model

Videotapes were used in a study by Barbara Melamed to help reduce children's dental fears. In group A, the children watched a film that gave a guided tour of a dentist's office. In group B, the children observed a film showing a young child going through a pleasant dental experience. The group B children, i.e. those who watched a model, were less afraid and better behaved than the group A children.

In another study, Melamed compared children who never had been to a dentist and observed the guided tour film (group A) with children who had previous dental experience and saw an irrelevant film (group B). The group A children became more disruptive in the dental office than the group B children. It may be that watching the film showing the dental office made the inexperienced children's fears more definitive (Hassett, 1978; Melamed et al., 1975).

3. Behavioral Rehearsal: Behavioral rehearsal involves having the patient practice the desired behavior until it no longer creates anxiety. The child can be shown and told what will occur at the next visit. He can also be encouraged to role play at home, e.g. play "dentist" and examine his mother's mouth. Fear is reduced if the child knows what to expect. This is also true for many adults. When a patient knows what to expect, the fear (especially fear of the unknown) usually diminishes (Box 5-7).

Box 5-7: Great Expectations

The authors conducted an experiment at Temple University that involved warning subjects of an impending stressor. When the subjects were prewarned about a stressful stimulus, i.e. the word *needle* would be said at a later time, their physiological and subjective responses were much less severe for most subjects than when they were stressed without warning. The physiological measures used were pulse rate, respiratory rate, and skin resistance levels and fluctuations. Paradoxically, there was a small number of subjects whose reactions were more severe when they were prewarned. For them, the anticipation apparently caused the stress levels to build up. For such individuals, it would be preferable if they were mentally somewhere else when undergoing dental treatment, to diminish their awareness of what would be occurring. Hence, the use of hypnosis might be of benefit for such individuals (Morse et al., 1978).

4. Systemic Desensitization: Systemic desensitization is a popular psychologic technique developed by Joseph Wolpe (Wolpe and Lazarus, 1966) that effectively controls most maladaptive anxiety. It can readily be adapted for dental anxiety (odontophobia). It involves teaching the patient a method of

deep relaxation while simultaneously presenting to the patient a graded series of increasingly anxiety-producing situations. These situations are based on the patient's particular anxieties or fears. For instance, if a patient is afraid of the drill, he might be asked to rate on an increasing scale his anxieties starting from approaching the office, to going to the reception room, to being seated, to being draped, to seeing the dentist wash his hands, to viewing the dental instruments, to feeling the explorer, and finally to having the drill inserted in his mouth. Then, while he is in a deep state of relaxation, imaginary scenes are described beginning with those that are least anxiety provoking, e.g. walking to the office, and ending with the most anxiety-provoking ones, e.g. drilling of a tooth. The effectiveness of the technique is based on the principle that "if a response inhibitory of anxiety can be made in the presence of anxiety-evoking stimuli, it will weaken the bond between these stimuli and the anxiety (Wolpe and Lazarus, 1966). This is interpreted to mean that it is impossible for anxiety and relaxation to exist simultaneously.

For the method to be effective, the person is usually taught progressive relaxation (Jacobson's method). While relaxed, the patient is first asked to visualize a non-anxiety-evoking situation, e.g. lying in the sun. Once he is well trained in the relaxation and visualization techniques, then the desensitization sessions are begun. It may take several visits for this method to be completely effective. The use of these common sense procedures at this relatively simple level is well within the capabilities of the dentist and his staff. It could be employed in the dental office setting by staff members, while not curtailing the dental chair time. Once the patient is desensitized, then dental treatment can be started at chairside, starting with the least anxiety-provoking procedures.

5. Forced Exposure: A rarely used method in dentistry is forced exposure. Yet, the procedure may be suited for the compliant patient who is directed to face the feared object while he is in a state of fear. Of course, the dentist should be comforting at the same time that he is direct, or the result might be to increase the patient's fear. For example, fear of the drill might

be overcome if the patient was made to face the drill, see it, hear it, and even feel it on his thumbnail.

Progressive Relaxation

Progressive relaxation is a method of deep relaxation devised by Edmund Jacobson in the United States in 1938. It is used by itself and as a means of inducing hypnosis. Progressive relaxation can be effective as a method of overcoming dental fears and anxieties. However, with this and the other methods of sedation and antianxiety control, it is imperative that the patient have full confidence in his doctor. The patient must be assured that technically he will be managed as well as possible. Positive reinforcement by other patients and staff members can help in this regard.

The actual technique of progressive relaxation is simple. As a rule, the patient lies down or sits inclined in a chair, e.g. contoured dental chair, closes his eyes, and alternately tenses and then relaxes a specific area of his body. The order or stages of relaxation are as follows: (1) the arms, (2) the legs, (3) concentration on breathing, (4) the forehead and the eyes, and (5) muscles of the larynx. Pain and anxiety tend to diminish when this relaxation method is used.

Autogenic Training

Deep relaxation and anxiety control may also be achieved by a method known as *autogenic training*. Developed by J. H. Schultz in Germany in 1932 and popularized by Wolfgang Luthe (1969), this technique is similar to autohypnosis. The patient sits inclined with eyes closed and concentrates on different parts of his body while responding to different mental cues for each particular area. For example, he thinks: "My right arm is heavy"; "My right arm is warm"; "My heart is beating calmly and regularly"; "My breathing is calm and regular"; "My abdomen is warm"; and "My forehead is cool."

The patient visualizes different autonomic responses that are conducive to decrease metabolism and increased relaxation. For instance, the sensations of heaviness and warmth of the limbs are particularly effective, as these sensations have been associated with muscular relaxation and increased blood flow. Autogenic training can be useful in overcoming dental fears and anxieties.

Hypnosis

Hypnosis is presumed to be an altered state of consciousness that is usually induced by the repetitive action of a constant stimulus. If the induction is facilitated by another person, it is *heterohypnosis;* if the induction is self-induced, it is *autohypnosis.* The attainment of a hypnotic state is related to (1) suggestibility (the ability to readily accept and act upon suggestions; (2) concentration; (3) motivation (generally the greater the desire, the better the chance of being hypnotized); (4) monotony (the more repetitive and ambiguous the stimuli, the more effective are they in inducing hypnosis); (5) imagination (the greater the visual imagery, the easier to achieve depth); and (6) the skill of the operator (not everyone has the ability nor the patience to be an effective hypnotist).

The hypnotized subject usually achieves varying degrees of relaxation, a focusing of concentration, subjective changes in body image, certain distortions of reality, and the ability to exert some control over autonomic nervous system functions. The individual is usually deeply relaxed, unless he has been given instructions to mentally engage in some task. Physiologically, when no mental task is given, the responses are those of deep relaxation; when a task is given, the opposite physiological responses are found (Box 5-8).

Box 5-8: The Two Sides of Hypnosis

In a study by the authors at Temple University, forty-eight subjects (Ss) were hypnotized while they were being simultaneously monitored (Fig. 5-2). The physiological measures used were blood pressure, pulse rate, brain wave patterns, muscle activity, and skin resistance. At a point when they were deeply relaxed, the Ss were given a mental task. They were told to imagine that their right hand was in an ice bucket. The physiological response levels and fluctuations were found to be in the direction of deep relaxation for relaxation-hypnosis and in the opposite direction for task-hypnosis (Morse et al., 1977).

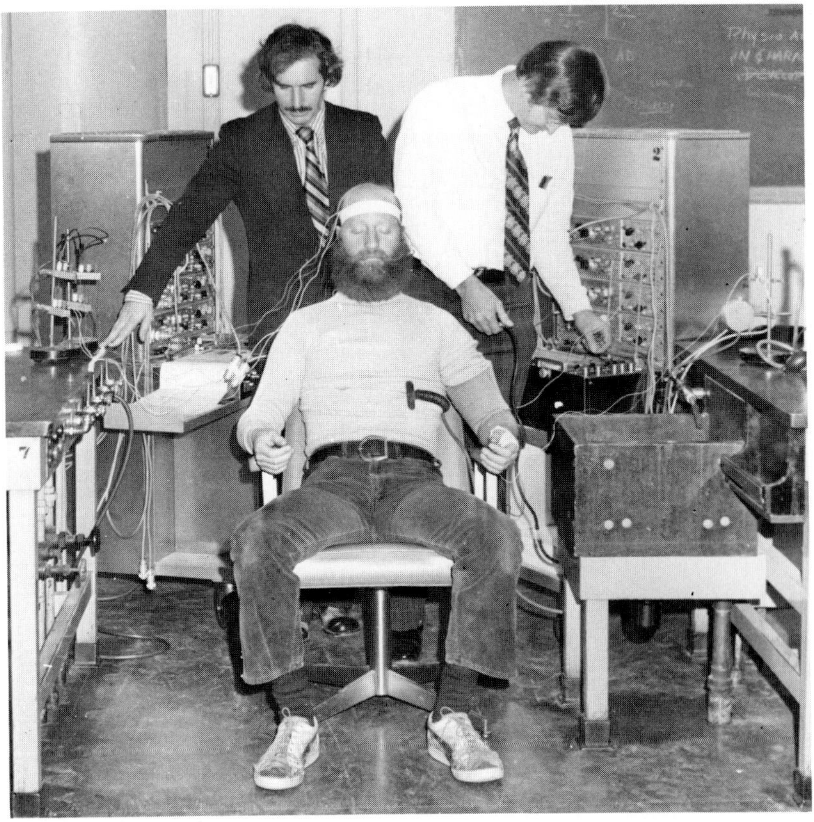

Figure 5-2. Wired up for hypnosis. Donald Morse (hypnotist) and John Martin (physiologist) are monitoring hypnotized subject, William Maher, Jr.

The various levels of hypnosis range from a slight relaxation to the somnambulistic state. There are two phases, the induction and the trance. The many methods of induction include (1) eye fixation (staring at an object till the eyes get tired and close); (2) breath counting; (3) eye rolling (keeping the head forward, looking upward with the eyes, and slowly closing the eyelids while still looking upward); and (4) meditation (constant, silent repetition of a sound). Once the eyes close, the trance is said to begin (Box 5-9).

Box 5-9: What Is This Thing Called Hypnosis?

Some authorities such as Theodore Barber (1974) do not agree that there is an actual trance or even a separate state as hypnosis. Barber's findings are that most, if not all, of the hypnotic phenomena can be produced while the subject is alert, if he is given sufficient motivation. However, most other authorities believe that hypnosis is a separate state, even though physiologically it cannot be distinguished clearly at this time (confirmed by the authors in a study at Temple University; Morse et al., 1977).

Once in the trance, the deeper the state, the more distinctive the phenomena that are generally observed. Some of the hypnotic phenomena are (1) arm levitation (arm or hand seemingly rises by itself); (2) eye catalepsy (eyelids cannot open); (3) limb rigidity (arms or legs become firm and immobile); (4) positive hallucinations (seeing objects that have no physical existence); (5) negative hallucinations (failure to perceive objects that exist); (6) positive and negative auditory, tactile, and olfactory hallucinations; (7) automatic writing (a hand appears to write by itself); (8) automatic movement (a hand or leg seemingly moves by itself); (9) amnesia (failure to recall what has occurred while in the trance); (10) analgesia (absence of perception of pain, a numb feeling or an "I don't care" attitude about the pain); (11) dissociation (feeling of being in two places at once or being able to separate the physical from the mental state); (12) dream induction (vivid dreams occur easily); (13) age regression or progression (ability to mentally go back or forward in time; and (14) posthypnotic suggestibility (doing things later, while presumably awake, that are suggested in the trance).

Only about 20 percent of the population has been found to achieve a deep-enough trance, i.e. somnambulism, to manifest most of these phenomena. However, for relief of dental anxiety and fear, it is generally not necessary to get the patient into a deep state, as relaxation takes place on a relatively light plane.

It is important that some of the myths surrounding hypnosis

be dispelled, since fear of hypnosis can dissuade some patients from agreeing to its use or becoming "good" subjects. These myths are now considered:

1. First, contrary to popular belief, there is no loss of control; all hypnosis is in actuality self-hypnosis. The patient does not do anything against his will or moral principles. However, being deeply relaxed and at ease, the patient may be more inclined to accept suggestions uncritically, and he might do something that he would not do when fully alert. Hence, since sexual feelings may be aroused, it is important that the male dentist-hypnotist have a female assistant present while hypnosis is being used (the reverse, of course, should hold for female dentist-hypnotists). Also, since the patient exercises less critical judgment while under hypnosis, it is possible that an unscrupulous operator could take advantage of the situation. Nonetheless, the authors and most authorities consider the practicing dentist to be ethical and moral, i.e. the health professional is to be distinguished from the amateurish "hypnotist," whose objectives might be quite different.

2. There is a widely held belief that a person can stay in a trance indefinitely, but a patient will eventually awaken even when all suggestions to do so are ignored at the time. Should the hypnotist die, the patient would still awaken. What usually happens is that the trance state converts into normal sleep. A quicker way to arouse the patient is to suggest to him that his bladder is full.

3. The ability to be hypnotized and control autonomic functions is a sign of a "strong will" and not a "weak will" as many people believe.

4. Anybody can be hypnotized if the motivation is strong enough and there is good rapport between the doctor and patient. Thus, patients in severe pain and experiencing anxiety are often the best subjects for hypnosis (Box 5-10).

Box 5-10: The Hypnotized Root Canal

In a clinical study, Donald Morse used a combination technique of meditation and hypnosis to overcome fear and anxiety and decrease pain for patients that required endodontic therapy. It was found that the patients who had unremitting pain and were extremely anxious were often the best hypnotic subjects; it was as if they were "grasping for straws." The fact that they were well motivated and that rapport was immediately established permitted rapid, effective hypnosis (Morse, 1976).

Although the methods of hypnosis appear to be simple and are attempted by some in a sophomoric way, e.g. having taken one course in introductory psychology, certain conditions should be met before its employment. First, obtaining a psychological profile, i.e. to assess ego strength, should be a preliminary step for any potential subject or patient in order to forestall any negative consequences. Also, dentists should not employ hypnosis unless they have been adequately trained. Courses are given by the American Society of Clinical Hypnosis (ASCH), the Society for Clinical and Experimental Hypnosis (SCEH), the American Society of Psychosomatic Dentistry and Medicine (ASPDM), and various dental schools.*

An example of a typical use of a current form of hypnosis is found in a case report drawn from an article by Morse (Box 5-12).

Box 5-12: Numbing Without Novocaine

Mr. V. M., aged 35 years, had an acute exacerbation of a chronic pulpitis of the upper left canine. Clinical manifestations included a severe toothache, tenderness to percussion and palpation, and sensitivity to heat and cold. The patient gave a history of having been successfully hypnotized 20 years earlier by a lay hypnotist. He had had no hypnotic experiences since that time. The patient objected to the feeling of numbness that one obtains from a local anesthetic injection and stated that he disliked the "needle." He said he would like to have his work performed under hypnosis.

*ASCH: 2400 East Devon Avenue, Suite 218, Des Plaines, Illinois 60018.
SCEH: Box 144, Liverpool, New York 13088.
ASPDM: 2802 Mermaid Avenue, Brooklyn, New York 11224.

Induction was obtained by the repetition of the word, "one." Hypno-analgesia was achieved by the suggestion of whole body and then facial numbness. This was then reinforced by glove anesthesia (bucket of ice method) with transference to the upper left canine and the surrounding gingival tissue. Deepening was achieved by the descending elevator method and the patient was instructed to take a pleasant trip. It took 10 minutes from eye closure to the beginning of treatment. A rubber dam was placed and saliva accumulation was prevented by suggesting to the patient that he keep his mouth dry. Access into the root canal was accomplished, and the vital and inflamed pulp was removed. The patient was told to stop the hemorrhage from the pulpal extirpation. Whether or not it was the result of the suggestion, bleeding was no problem. The canal was instrumented, irrigated, and filled. The patient was then given a posthypnotic suggestion that anesthesia would last in the tooth and gingiva for a half-hour, after which the area would feel normal.

At the conclusion of the treatment, the patient was told that he would awaken at his own pace, feeling completely relaxed with no discomfort.

The patient commented upon awakening that he had felt no pain at all; he said that he had felt a slight amount of pressure, but it was not bothersome. He said that it was as if it had occurred to someone else that he had been observing. The patient stated that the area was still numb, but he felt fine and thoroughly enjoyed the experience. He said he took a pleasant trip but declined to describe it. The patient remained numb for about a half-hour and had no postoperative discomfort. (From D. R. Morse: Use of a Meditative State for Hypnotic Induction in the Practice of Endodontics, *Oral Surgery, 41*:664, 1976. Reprinted with permission of the C. V. Mosby Co., St. Louis.)

With the patient described in the case report, no local anesthetic was used. However, for most patients, hypnosis should not be relied upon for complete analgesia. Rather, it should be used to overcome apprehension and allow for reduced local anesthetic doses and painless local anesthetic injections. Effective use of hypnosis also results in relaxed oral musculature and permits the patient to take a "mental trip" away from the dental office. With some patients, other benefits can occur, such as decreased salivation, decreased bleeding, inhibition of gagging, decreased postoperative discomfort, and more rapid healing.

*Meditation**

> Meditation is [presumed to be] a self-activated altered state of consciousness which is induced by the repetitive action of a constant stimulus [Box 5-13]. The stimulus may be external, internal or physical. As the result of repeated stimulation, an individual, without trying, achieves varying degrees of relaxation, subjective changes in body image, certain distortions of reality and the ability to decrease autonomic nervous system functions. In addition, the subject appears to attain an improved understanding of himself and may consider that an expansion of consciousness or a higher state of consciousness has occurred. [Morse, 1977a]

Box 5-13: The Mystical Sound of Silence by D.M.

With poetic license, impressions and reflections of a first mantra-type meditation are presented.

A sound is heard
An eerie word
I close my eyes
I hear its vibes

I speak it softly
I feel it gently
And my limbs lighten
As my thoughts quicken

Then the sound repeats
In rhythmic beats

*A discussion of the realm of higher states of consciousness is beyond the scope of this book.

And my mind retreats
From its daily feats

Thoughts come and go
My breathing's slow
And the sound repeats
With leisure beats

And my toes tingle
As new thoughts mingle
And the sound repeats
With lulling beats

My mind is still
Without a will
Then the sound repeats
With quiet beats

And then no mind
No thoughts to find
And the sound repeats
In silent beats

A yawn, a sigh
A stretch, a cry
Then the sound retreats
And my mind's at peace

The most popular method of meditation is mantra meditation, in which a sound, word, or phrase is silently repeated while the subject sits partially inclined with eyes closed in a relaxed position (Box 5-14). Transcendental Meditation (TM) is the most well-known meditation technique.

Box 5-14: The Secret Word

A mantra is an ancient Sanskrit sound, word, or phrase that is specifically chosen, according to the ancient Vedic tradition, for its soothing, salutary, mystical, or religious meaning. With TM, mantras are chosen from the list assembled by Maharishi Mahesh Yogi (the founder of TM). A selected mantra is assigned by a TM teacher to each initiate during a semi-religious mystical ceremony.

Physiological studies have shown that mantra meditation can induce physiological changes suggestive of deep relaxation (Bloomfield, 1962). However, contrary to earlier findings, TM is not unique in the changes that are produced. Several studies have shown that similar changes can be induced during deep relaxation, relaxation-hypnosis, autogenic training, simple-word meditation, and religious meditation (Benson et al., 1974; Morse et al., 1977; Walrath and Hamilton, 1975; Box 5-15).

Box 5-15: All "Trips" Lead to Nirvana

The authors were involved in a study at Temple University in which no significant physiological differences were found between relaxation, relaxation-hypnosis, simple-word meditation, and TM. The physiological measures used were pulse rate, respiratory rate, muscle activity, brain wave patterns, blood pressure, and skin resistance levels and fluctuations. Subjectively, the participants reported similar feelings of deep relaxation, euphoria, and dissociation for relaxation-hypnosis, simple-word meditation, and TM. However, relaxation was found not to be as effective as the others (Morse et al., 1977).

Studies have also shown that meditation decreases pain and anxiety, and it can effectively be used to control dental fears, anxieties, and pain (Morse, 1976; Morse and Hildebrand, 1976). An example of the use of meditation for hypnosis was drawn from the case report presented in the previous section. The senior author used meditation alone to induce relaxation and decrease pain for himself while undergoing periodontal surgical procedures (Fig. 5-3). Other patients have also used meditation alone and have reported that it reduces anxiety (Morse, 1976; Morse and Hildebrand, 1976).

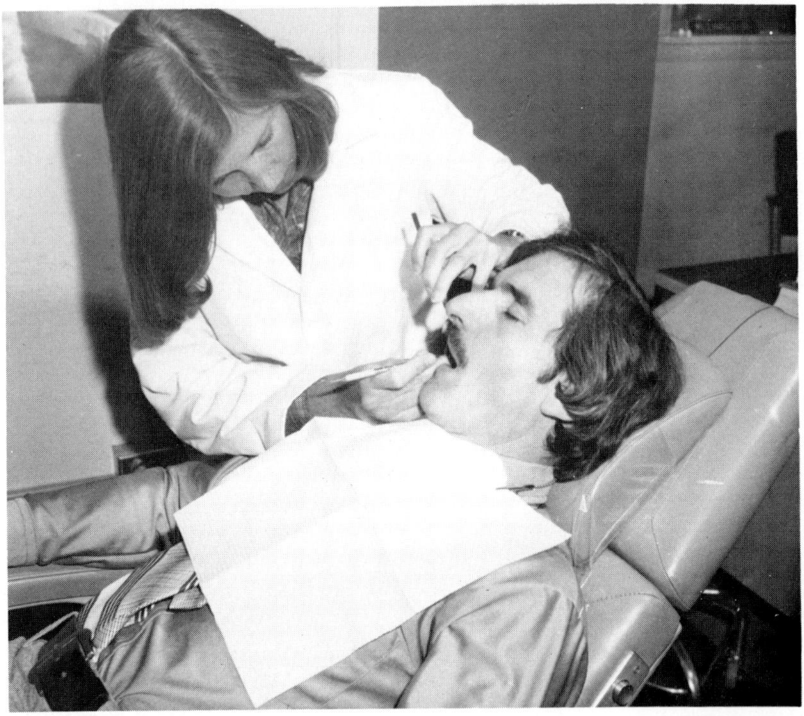

Figure 5-3. Meditation and periodontics. Donald Morse is using meditation for relaxation and pain control, while Carol Hildebrand (periodontist) is performing periodontal treatment. (From D. R. Morse and C. N. Hildebrand, Case Report: Use of TM in Periodontal Therapy, *Dental Survey, 52(11):* 36, 1976. Courtesy of *Dental Survey* and Harcourt Brace Jovanovich, Inc., New York, New York.)

As the result of the investigation and use of hypnosis and meditation by the authors, a combined technique has been devised. It can be used by patients while they are being treated. It permits decreased anxiety, painless injections, reduced doses of local anesthetic, relaxed oral musculature, and allows the patient to take a pleasant "mental trip" away from the office. The combined technique is also an excellent way for the dentist to cope with the stressors of dental practice (*see* Chap. 6).

It generally only takes a few minutes to teach meditation-hypnosis to patients, and the benefits are well worth the time and effort involved. The technique is described in Box 5-16 for use with patients; the discussion about time is not relevant, except that the patient should not present himself for treatment immediately after eating.

Box 5-16: Traveling Through Time and Space

Meditation-hypnosis is generally practiced for a 20-30 minute period prior to dinner. If you are very hungry or thirsty, you should take a small snack and then wait an hour. If you do not have the time before dinner, wait two hours after dinner and then begin. Experience has shown that an empty or full stomach interferes with proper meditation-hypnosis. If you can accustom yourself, it is also advantageous to practice the technique prior to breakfast. Before beginning at either time, it is important to empty your bladder and/or colon as fullness of either impedes relaxation. When you are ready, go to a quiet darkened room where you will not be distracted (away from the telephone, radio, etc.). The room should be clean and well ventilated with a moderate temperature. Dust, cold, warmth, and drafts all impede relaxation. Now pick a comfortable chair and you are ready to begin.

Sit partially inclined (horizontal position can induce sleep) while keeping your feet on the ground, uncrossed. Loosen your clothes; remove your shoes, watch, rings, glasses, etc. Place your hands, also uncrossed, on your lap or the sides of the chair. These are done to decrease external pressure on your body.

Now inhale, exhale, close your eyes, and remain quiet for about a minute. Then, silently repeat a word (in clinical and research studies, it was found that most people preferred words with neutral or pleasant connotations such as, "one," "love," and "flower"). The word is repeated at any pace (e.g., to your heart beat or respiratory rate). After a while thoughts may intrude. They should be completed, but when you realize it, you then return to the repetition of the word. In time, the word may appear distorted, but don't concern yourself.

While meditating, mentally concentrate on your toes. Think about them and then relax them. Continue concentrating and relaxing with various muscle groups until you reach the scalp. Then proceed internally, relax your lungs, intestines, blood flow, etc. After a while, you may feel a warm, tingling, floating feeling throughout your body.

Now is the time to take a mental trip. Suggest to yourself a lovely, quiet place. It could be a lake, a brook, a stream, the beach, or the mountains. But it should be a place you want to go. The more engrossed you are with the trip, the easier it is to forget your word. But don't worry. However, if you feel you are becoming alert, then return to the word. In time, you may forget the trip and the word and have a "blank mind." This is the deepest state and most people find it extremely pleasant.

Keep a watch nearby so that you can glance at it occasionally. Don't use an alarm clock, for you don't want to be jolted. After about 20 minutes, begin to arouse yourself. Take about 1-2 minutes to gradually return to normal. Stretch and slowly open your eyes. You should feel alert and refreshed. If you feel a little light-headed, take a little longer to awaken. (From D. R. Morse: Variety, Exercise, Meditation Can Relieve Practice Stress, *Dental Student, 56(3)*:26, 1977. Courtesy of *Dental Student* and Stevens Publishing Corporation.)

Biofeedback

It was formerly believed in the United States that autonomic nervous system responses could never be brought under voluntary control. In light of experiments performed in the Soviet Union (Ivanov-Smolensky, 1954) and later in the United States by Neal Miller (1977) working with rats, it was shown that autonomic nervous system responses could be voluntarily controlled and this control could be selective, e.g. lowering pulse rate while simultaneously raising blood pressure. As a result of these findings, the technique of biofeedback came into prominance.

Biofeedback is a method that uses various procedures and instruments to teach individuals voluntary control over heretofore involuntary processes, such as heart rate, blood pressure, brain wave production, muscle activity, vasodilation, vasoconstriction, and skin resistance levels and fluctuations.

With the use of the relaxation response, e.g. progressive relaxation, autogenic training, relaxation-hypnosis, and meditation, there is no selectivity in the autonomic changes. For instance, generally there are decreases found in heart rate, respiratory rate, muscle activity, blood pressure, and fluctuations in skin resistance, i.e. decreased sweat gland activity. However, with biofeedback, each one of these physiological responses could be selectively altered.

There are two aspects to biofeedback control. The first is awareness; the patient must be made aware of the physiological activity by a specific signal (visual or auditory). The second is action; once the patient is aware of the activity, he must change it in the desired direction. In order to change the activity, the patient must use his own specific technique. For instance, he could use self-hypnosis or work by trial and error. The patient is made aware of the change in physiological activity by an alteration of the signal. For example, one technique is to attach electrodes from the biofeedback monitor to the hand in order to detect skin resistance levels and changes. A second connection goes to an FM radio. When the electrodes are first connected, there is no sound coming from the radio. When the individual is asked to increase skin resistance level (decreased sympathetic nervous system activity produces this effect), he might try to effect this change by self-hypnosis. Without being fully conscious of what was happening physiologically, he would know he was being successful when he heard music coming from the speaker. The louder the music being played, the greater would be the increase in skin resistance. However, if the music stops, then the patient would have a way of knowing that he was not changing the skin resistance in the desired direction.

In medicine and psychology, there are various types of biofeedback instruments that are adapted for use with heart rate, skin resistance (galvanic skin response or GSR), brain wave patterns (specifically trying to attain high levels of alpha), blood flow (to decrease tension or migraine headaches), and muscle activity (to try to reduce microvoltage output of muscles, known as electromyographic activity or EMG). In dentistry, the most popular technique is the use of EMG feedback.

Andres Cannistraci has pioneered in the development of this technique. A typical machine is shown in Figure 5-4. The electrodes are placed in a band that is fitted over the patient's frontalis muscles (Fig. 5-5). As the muscles relax, the electromyographic activity decreases (and vice versa with increased muscle contraction). With these changes in muscle activity, there are visual changes displayed on the machine dial, and the patient hears or fails to hear a beeper tone (depends upon muscular contraction or relaxation).

Since a biofeedback machine is not inexpensive and its use takes time, one may question its value, especially when meditation and hypnosis require no machinery and often can be performed more rapidly. One answer is that some patients cannot get as deeply relaxed with hypnosis and meditation as they can with biofeedback assistance (Box 5-17).

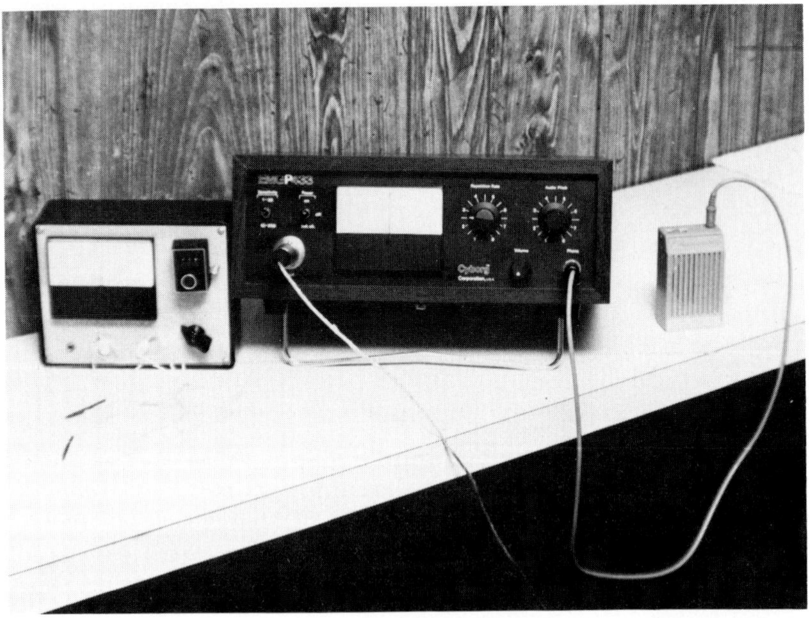

Figure 5-4. A typical EMG biofeedback unit used in dentistry, the electromyographic biofeedback instrument EMGP433, manufactured by Cyborg Corporation. (Courtesy of Dr. Andres Cannistraci, New York, New York.)

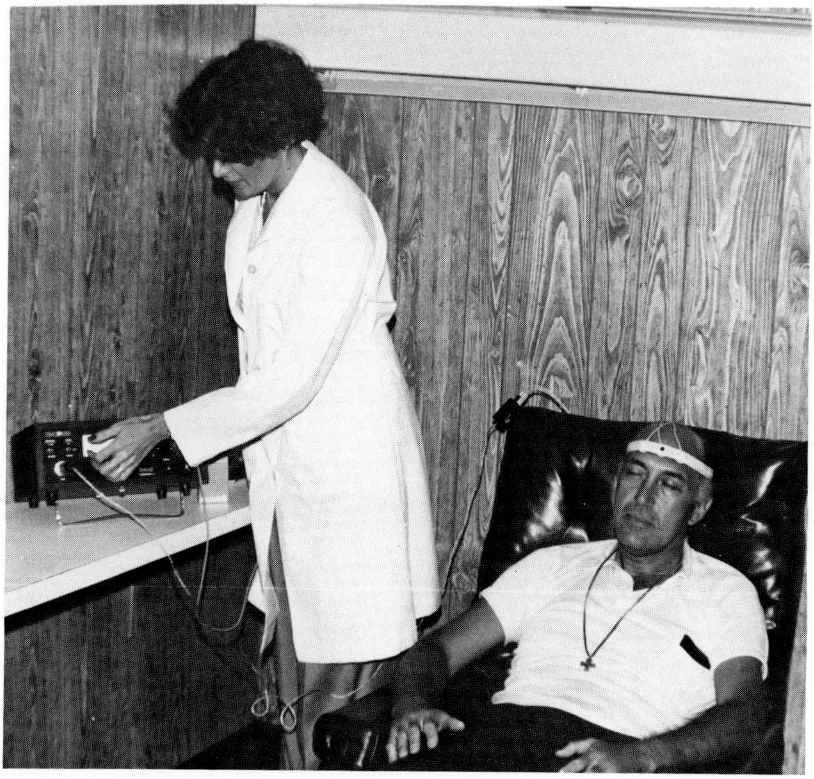

Figure 5-5. Wired for biofeedback. A patient is being prepared for biofeedback-assisted relaxation by biofeedback trainer, Judith Proctor. (Courtesy of Dr. Andres Cannistraci, New York, New York.)

Box 5-17: Biofeedback Triumphs!

In a clinical study comparing biofeedback with relaxation techniques, it was shown that within a single session subjects who use EMG biofeedback were able to achieve lower levels of muscle activity than those subjects who were instructed in relaxation without feedback. It is thought that when subjects can be made aware of their level of relaxation (by signals), they can become more deeply relaxed than when they relax without any feedback to show them how "deep" they are (Budyznski and Stoyva, 1973).

Another reason for the use of biofeedback is that even a dentist who may not be an effective hypnotist can readily use biofeedback to help patients relax. Some practitioners use biofeedback in the beginning to put the control of the relaxation literally in the hands of the patient. When the patients become proficient, then the relaxation method is used alone without the aid of the machine.

Audioanalgesia

Audioanalgesia was a popular technique in the late 1960s that utilized music and a "white" sound (where all frequencies have equal probability) in an effort to block dental pain. The patient wore stereo headphones and listened to semiclassical music. When a painful sensation was felt or anticipated the patient turned a dial that increased the intensity of the white noise. Apparently, the effectiveness was based on the then unknown gate-control theory of pain, in which activation of large nerve fibers (stimulated by the white noise) prevented the central transmission of the smaller pain-producing nerve fibers (Melzack and Wall, 1965). This technique was not too successful, and after an initial prominance, it soon fell into disuse. Still, it was observed that the use of the stereo music had a calming effect on many patients. But when the dentist chose the music, the results were not always predictable. Permitting patients to choose the type of music was found to be a better technique because, although semiclassical music was usually preferred, occasionally some teenagers, for example, actually relaxed better with hard rock.

A new technique developed by Philip Rich (1977), combines patient-selected stereo music with a foot-activated switch that allows for necessary conversation between the staff and the patient. An advantage of headphones is that the patient can take a "mental trip" and he does not hear the sound of the dental engine. Stereophonic music can be combined with hypnosis, meditation, or conscious sedation. Robert Atterbury (1974) used stereo headphones to give patients taped relaxation instructions. That method could easily be combined with music once the patient had achieved the necessary level of relaxation. Whether music is used as background in the entire office or individually in a headset, there is no doubt that music can decrease patient anxiety and fear.

Massage

There are certain manipulative techniques that can greatly relax an apprehensive patient. However, they are now rarely used in dentistry. There are two probable reasons for this situation. Historically, one of the roles of the barber-dentist was to massage the neck as well as the scalp. To dissociate themselves from barbering is one of the reasons why dentists have discontinued massage. Another reason is related to the "laying on of hands." Touching of the patient has sexual overtones, and dentists now have great fears of malpractice actions. Nevertheless, there is a place for massage and vibration in the dental setting. To avoid the problems associated with touching, dentists can use dental chairs with built-in vibrators. Another approach could be to allow the female assistants to perform the neck or facial muscle massage. Portable electrical units are excellent and can also be used by the dental staff for self-relaxation.

Summary

As can be seen, there are many effective relaxation methods. The important aspect with the drugless approaches is the approach to the patient, not the particular technique that is used. The dentist and staff should be gentle, positive, empathetic, and patient. With this kind of approach, most of the techniques can be successfully used.

The Drug Methods

Introduction

Although the previously described drugless techniques can be quite effective in reducing anxiety and increasing relaxation, they are not as predictable as methods in which drugs are used. However, the disadvantages of drug-related methods are that all drugs have undesirable side effects and can have dangerous interactions with other drugs the patients may be taking. Also, some drugs may occasionally react paradoxically; for example, barbiturates may cause excitement rather than relaxation. As discussed later, a balance can be achieved when drug use is decreased as the result of the combination of psychologic relaxation methods with drugs. Drug techniques vary from the use of simple placebos to general anesthesia in the hospital O. R. As these methods have been exhaustively covered in many publications (*see* References), only their general applicability to anxiety reduction is covered. Sedatives and tranquilizers and the placebo effect are first discussed.

Oral Drugs and Placebo Effect

There are three basic categories of drugs that are used to overcome patient apprehension: (1) barbiturate sedatives, (2) nonbarbiturate sedatives, and (3) antianxiety agents (minor tranquilizers). These drugs do not have an analgesic effect, and if the patient is in pain, analgesics such as aspirin, acetaminophen, e.g. Tylenol®, codeine, and Percodan® should also be used. Sedatives act by affecting the cerebral cortex; antianxiety agents selectively depress the subcortical areas. Drugs of the latter kind cause less of a decrease in mental alertness than do the sedatives; they also may arrest aggressive actions. Patients who take antianxiety agents should be cautioned against driving, since these drugs can cause lethargy or drowsiness. Patients who take sedatives must not be allowed to drive, since these drugs cause drowsiness. These contraindications are not found with the use of meditation and hypnosis, and this is one reason why these may be more appropriate.

In increased doses, sedatives act as hypnotics (sleep induction). However with some active children, paradoxical excitation reactions can occur (especially with the barbiturates). Hence, with children, comedication with nitrous oxide-oxygen might be more effective. Both antianxiety agents and sedatives can be used intravenously for control of apprehension. Patients who are already taking depressants or antihistamines should be given decreased doses of sedatives or antianxiety agents, since there are additive effects and dangerous respiratory depression could occur.

Part of the effectiveness of all drugs is related to the placebo effect. *Placebo* is a term derived from the Latin verb, *placere,* meaning "to please." It is used to describe any therapy or drug that is used for a specific effect without having any known pharmacologic or therapeutic effect for the specific condition being treated. Placebos work best when the patient has a high level of anxiety and when other indicators of stress levels are high. Placebos also work well when the patients expect or anticipate relief. Suggestibility is a factor. When the practitioner conveys enthusiasm for the effectiveness of the drug, it generally works better. This is also true of the positive pronouncements by the staff relating to the effectiveness of the therapy.

Placebos have a real effect; they probably work on the autonomic nervous system in much the same manner as hypnosis and biofeedback. As it is considered unethical not to inform the patient about the drug being prescribed, simple placebos cannot be used therapeutically. However, the placebo effect enhances the effectiveness of sedatives and antianxiety drugs. Hence, the dentist and his staff should be enthusiastic when prescribing drugs, and then the dose can probably be reduced. In Table 5-I, a summary of useful sedatives and antianxiety agents is given.

Local Anesthesia

There are several methods to allay apprehension and diminish the perception of pain when local anesthetic injections are to be used. First, preinjection use of techniques such as hypnosis, meditation, audioanalgesia, conscious sedation, and drug premedication can allow for relatively painless injections. The patient is usually on a mental trip and is not aware of the actual penetration of the needle. A second method is to use an

Table 5-I

TYPICAL SEDATIVES AND ANTIANXIETY AGENTS*

Agent	*Category*	*Usual Dose*
Pentobarbital (Nembutal®)	Sedative	30 mg the night before the visit; 60 mg one-half hour before the visit
Secobarbital (Seconal®)	Sedative	50 mg the night before the visit 50 mg one-half hour before the visit
Ethinamate (Valmid®)	Sedative	One to two tablets (500 mg to 1 gr) the night before the visit; one tablet one-half hour before the visit
Chloral hydrate (Noctec®)	Sedative	500 mg (in syrup) one-half hour before the visit
Chlordiazepoxide (Librium)	Antianxiety agent	One capsule (5 mg) morning and evening starting two days before the visit; two capsules one hour before the visit
Diazepam (Valium)	Antianxiety agent	One capsule (5 mg) morning and evening starting two days before the visit; two capsules one hour before the visit
Hydroxyzine (Atarax®, Vistaril®)	Antianxiety agent	50 mg the night before the visit; 50 mg one-half hour before the visit
Meprobamate (Equanil, Miltown)	Antianxiety agent	One tablet (200 or 400 mg) four times daily beginning three days before the visit

*From D. R. Morse: *Clinical Endodontology: A Comprehensive Guide to Diagnosis, Treatment and Prevention,* 1974. Courtesy of Charles C Thomas, Publisher, Springfield, Illinois.

effective topical anesthetic. A third technique is the use of pressure anesthesia, e.g. Syri-jet®.

Even if none of these techniques are used, painless injections can still be achieved. First, one should always use the finest disposable needle available. In that way, the insertion and penetration are relatively painless. Second, in order to decrease apprehension, the needle should be kept out of sight. The patient could be asked to close his eyes and breathe through his nose while the injection is given. If the patient's eyes are open, fear is intensified. As one college student stated, "I have an abiding distrust of needles, especially when the person wielding one is hiding it behind his back" (Hassett, 1978). An interesting anecdote with reference to keeping one's eyes closed is related in Box 5-18.

Box 5-18: Open Your Mouth and Close Your Eyes

> A dental student presented himself to the junior author (M.F.) with the problem of having to administer a local anesthetic injection to patients with his own eyes open. He had been conditioned by his parents to always take local anesthetic injections for his own dental treatments with his eyes closed. This conflict prevented his giving local anesthetic injections while his own eyes stayed open. Resolution through deconditioning permitted the student to fulfill his dental school requirements.

Another way to decrease pain and anxiety is to apply lip pressure with one hand while simultaneously delivering the injection with the other hand. When giving a palatal injection, pressure with a dental mirror on the palatal mucosa can decrease the pain of the injection. In these techniques, the application of pressure activates the large nerve fibers, which mask the effects of the smaller pain-producing nerve fibers, i.e. according to the gate-control theory. It is believed that anxiety keeps the pain gate open.

To decrease apprehension, it is essential that the anesthetic be effective. Therefore, an adequate dose of the correct anesthetic must be delivered to the anatomically proper position (Morse, 1974).

Conscious Sedation Techniques

There are two basic conscious sedation, i.e. psychosedation, techniques. These are (1) nitrous oxide-oxygen relative analgesia (inhalation sedation); and (2) intravenous sedation (I.V. sedation, chemanalgesia, and parenteral conscious sedation). Inhalation sedation is the most popular and safest. I.V. sedation is the most effective but has some hazards.

1. INHALATION SEDATION: Nitrous oxide-oxygen relative anal-

gesia is a method of sedation, tranquilization, and analgesia in which a small rubber nosepiece is used for the delivery of the gaseous mixture (Fig. 5-6). It is more effective and reliable than oral sedatives and antianxiety agents but less effective than I.V. sedation. Training is less detailed than is required for the use of I.V. sedation, and monitoring of the patient is simpler. Nevertheless, no one should use this method unless he has taken an approved course.*

Generally, when the patient's mouth begins to close, the

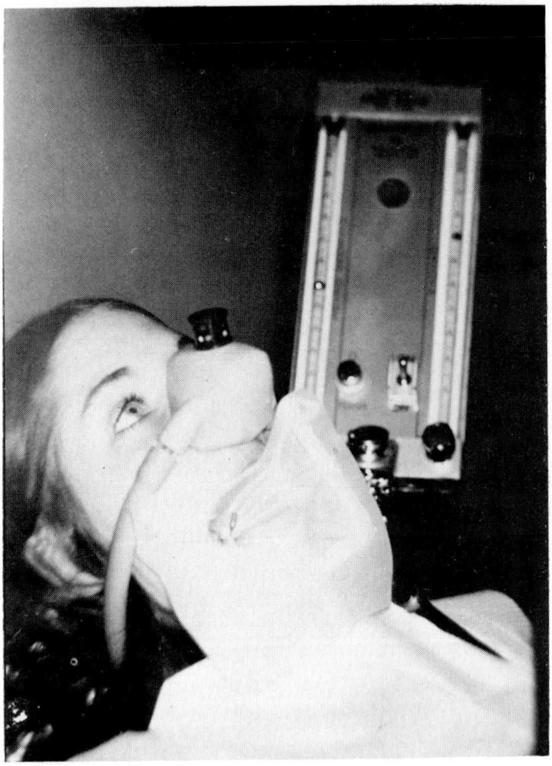

Figure 5-6. Nitrous oxide-oxygen relative analgesia in use with rubber dam in position. (From D. R. Morse, *Clinical Endodontology: A Comprehensive Guide to Diagnosis, Treatment and Prevention,* 1974. Courtesy of Charles C Thomas, Publisher, Springfield, Illinois.)

*Courses on inhalation sedation are given by many dental schools and dental societies.

patient is too deep. With the newer machines, no less than 2.5 liters min. of oxygen can be delivered, and if the oxygen supply runs out, the nitrous oxide automatically cuts off, i.e. the fail-safe system. The hoses, valves, and settings are also specific for each gas and cannot be transposed.

Side effects are rare and include nausea, vomiting, and persisting euphoria. Most patients feel pleasantly relaxed or even exhilarated. After being administered pure oxygen for a few minutes, patients usually can drive home unaided. Occasionally, patients who fear masks or loss of control may feel trapped when inhalation sedation is used. For these individuals, a different modality should be used.

Since with the use of inhalation sedation a degree of analgesia is obtained, it is often possible to reduce or even eliminate local anesthesia. Use of inhalation sedation with hypnosis and/or meditation is effective, and usually the dose of the nitrous oxide can be greatly reduced. Use of inhalation sedation with oral sedatives generally results in decreased doses of both, and, therefore, there is less danger of toxic results.

One recently discovered potential problem with the use of inhalation sedation is the toxicity of the drugs to the staff from gas leaks through the nosepiece and hoses. Since there are now mechanisms available that can monitor and remove waste gases, this problem may be minimized (Voss and Shimoda, 1977).

2. I.V. Sedation: I.V. sedation is the use of chemical agents injected intravenously for the purpose of psychosedation and varying degrees of analgesia. Various types of drugs can be used, but the safest, most effective drug is diazepam (Valium). Valium gives relief of anxiety and produces sedation, partial analgesia, muscle relaxation, and amnesia (at times). Although I.V. sedation gives the greatest degree of sedation, as compared to psychological, oral, or inhalation techniques, it also demands the greatest amount of caution. Under no circumstances should I.V. sedation be used unless the dentist has had adequate training. One-week dental society and dental school-sponsored courses are available. This is the minimum post-

graduate training that a dentist should have.

Most patients have pleasurable sensations and a feeling of euphoria from the use of I.V. sedation. Side effects are rare, but dentists using this modality should be well trained in resuscitation, and there should be adequate recovery room facilities. Patients should not drive home unaided.

As with inhalation sedatives, the dose of local anesthesia can usually be reduced, and combined I.V. sedation with hypnosis or meditation allows for a reduced dose of Valium. The use of I.V. sedation with inhalation sedation also allows for a reduced dose of Valium.

General Anesthesia

With general anesthesia, the patient is rendered unconscious. As a result, the maximum degree of sedation, muscle relaxation, analgesia, and amnesia occurs. However, it is the most dangerous method and should only be employed by a dentist who has had a minimum of a one-year hospital and dental school anesthesia residency. General anesthesia should only be used in a hospital or in an office thoroughly set up for its use.

There are various ways of achieving general anesthesia with the most popular being (1) Brevital® sodium with nitrous oxide-oxygen, (2) Brevital sodium with Demerol®, HCl and nitrous oxide-oxygen, (3) Brevital sodium with Fluothane® and nitrous oxide-oxygen, (4) Brevital sodium with Nisentil® and nitrous oxide-oxygen, and Pentothal® sodium with nitrous oxide-oxygen.

General anesthesia is rarely used to overcome fear. However, it is indicated in the following cases: (1) patients who have uncontrollable fear or anxiety; (2) patients who are debilitated and hospitalized; (3) patients who have acute pain that cannot be relieved by any other method; and (4) patients who are either severely retarded, have cerebral palsy, are emotionally disturbed, or are psychotic.

It must be realized that the use of general anesthesia does not train patients to overcome their anxieties and fears (Box 5-19).

Box 5-19: Holding Down the General

The senior author (D.M.) has been practicing in a dental office in which general anesthesia is employed. Prior to D.M.'s entrance into the practice, there were many fearful patients who elected to have their dentistry done under general anesthesia. Since D.M. has been associated in the practice, hypnosis and meditation have been introduced as alternative methods. As a result, in the last two years, the use of general anesthesia has decreased by almost 40 percent.

Summary

Since there are several drug-related ways to allay anxiety and increase relaxation, the choice of the method depends upon the doctor, the patient, and particular circumstances. Generally, one should use the safest method possible that produces the desired therapeutic effect. From the previous discussion, it can be surmised that combining psychological approaches with drug-related methods can yield effective results and at the same time allow for a decrease in the required dose of the drugs. With this combined approach, the dentist can achieve reliable and positive results with a great margin of safety.

TREATING STRESS-RELATED ORAL DISEASES

Introduction

The stress-related oral diseases range from caries through NUG, bruxism, myofascial pain-dysfunction syndrome, and recurrent aphthous stomatitis. For each disease, there are well-known specific treatments, and thus these need not be covered in depth here. There are also nonspecific therapies related to the underlying stress. For the stress aspects, treatment includes behavior modification, hypnosis, meditation, biofeedback, anti-anxiety agents, and exercise. The discussion begins with caries and endodontic diseases.

Caries and Endodontic Diseases

As incidence of caries is partly related to stress-induced decreased salivation, drugs to increase salivation may be used. However, since there are other parasympathetic effects, these drugs must be used with extreme caution. The most useful drug is pilocarpine (usual dose, 5 mg orally).

To prevent stress-related flare-ups such as aerodontalgia and periapical pain and swelling, teeth with inflamed pulps should be treated endodontically, and the endodontic treatment should not have imperfections.

Periodontal Diseases

Since stressors, including physical proximity, are important components in the etiology of NUG, methods of reducing stressful occurrences should be employed. Overcrowding should be avoided (Box 5-20).

Box 5-20: Too Close For Comfort II

> A recent study showed that overcrowding, such as that occurring in subways, causes increases in heart rate, blood pressure, respiratory rate, and palmar sweating. Hence, there are physiological as well as psychological reasons to avoid crowding (Editorial: Feeling Tense, 1977).

Techniques such as meditation, hypnosis, and biofeedback can be used to teach the patient to regularly elicit the relaxation response. It is also essential to treat the diseases locally by scaling, curettage, and lavages, etc.

Clenching, Bruxism, and Myofascial Pain-Dysfunction Syndrome

Of all the stress-related oral diseases, clenching, bruxism, and myofascial pain-dysfunction syndrome are the conditions that have received the greatest variety of treatments, including stress-reducing methods.

Clenching and Bruxism

Clenching and bruxism are stress reactions that can be managed by making the patient aware of what he is doing and then help him to stop, treat, and prevent the condition. Drugs that are used include Valium, Librium®, and meprobamate (Miltown® and Equanil®). These antianxiety agents are also muscle relaxants and can help prevent the masticatory muscle contractions that occur during clenching and bruxism. Ethyl chloride spray has been used effectively to achieve muscle relaxation (Travell, 1960).

Nondrug methods are also quite effective. Palatal appliances such as nite-guards are used. The rationale is that the appliance stops the teeth from occluding, thereby relieving muscle spasms and preventing the teeth from grinding. Another technique is to teach the patient isotonic and isometric jaw exercises that help relax muscles that have been in a state of tension.

Leonard Zeldow (1976) described a method of habit retraining in which the attempt is to train the central nervous system to subconsciously relax the oral, facial, and cranial musculature even while the patient may still be under mental stress. The tongue is also taught to relax and be limp to help prevent contact of the teeth. The primary muscle groups that are trained are the frontalis (of the forehead), the tongue, and the masseter. The rationale is based on the fact that contraction of the frontalis causes the masseter and other muscle groups of the head and neck to contract, whereas relaxation of the frontalis causes relaxation of the scalp, neck, and upper body muscles. The patient practices this relaxation technique repeatedly until a more desirable habit takes over.

Meditation, autogenic training, and hypnosis are being used to induce the relaxation response and hopefully decrease anxiety and muscle tension. However, of all the nondrug methods, the most popular has been EMG biofeedback. Andres Cannistraci (1976) has described the technique used for the bruxism patient (Box 5-22).

Box 5-22: Biofeedbacking Bruxism

> With the bruxing patient, electrodes in a headband retainer are placed over the frontalis muscles of the forehead since these are excellent barometers of a patient's relaxation level and earphones are placed over the patient's ears to block out the sound of everything but the beeper. The patient has been shown the instrument panel and a needle which moves to the right when he clenches. The patient has been told that the beeper's tone rises in pitch whenever his jaw muscle activity increases and becomes lower when he relaxes and has pleasant feelings. In this way auditory and visual signals challenge the patient to lower the beeper tone and make the needle move toward the left.
>
> Biofeedback provides a patient with a skill and a feeling of contentment when using a feedback instrument. As he learns to lower the beeper's tone, he gets a feeling of accomplishment which, in turn, motivates him to achieve even greater relaxation. Secondly, as the stressed and bruxing patient relaxes, he experiences relief from tension and stress-induced muscle activity (Cannistraci, 1976).

If none of the methods help, it may be that the clenching and bruxism are caused by deep-seated emotional problems. In that case, psychological or psychiatric help is indicated (Box 5-23).

Box 5-23: Liberating Bruxism

> Cinotti and Grieder have another approach for bruxing women: "Movements like 'women's lib' may help too. Liberation may permit women to vent aggressive tendencies more openly and freely, and this may reduce the incidence of bruxism (Editorial: Mysterious Headaches, 1976). The concept might also be, "If the mouth is busy talking, it hasn't the time to brux."

Myofascial Pain-Dysfunction Syndrome

The treatments for myofascial pain-dysfunction syndrome are varied. Methods that have been or are used include (1) occlusal equilibration; (2) nite-guards; (3) splints; (4) corticosteroid injections into the temporomandibular joint or the masticatory muscles; (5) hyaluronidase or sclerosing solution injections into the joint; (6) local anesthetic or ethyl chloride injections into the masticatory muscles; (7) drug therapy, including placebos, antidepressants, antianxiety agents and sedatives; and (8) nondrug methods, including progressive relaxation, autogenic training, hypnosis, meditation, electrical (transcutaneous) stimulation, acupuncture, and biofeedback.

One treatment that has been well documented is the use of EMG biofeedback. Electrodes are generally placed on either the temporalis, masseter, or frontalis muscles. The technique is similar to that described on page 168.

Psychological counseling may also be necessary for cases that do not respond to the previously described methods.

Tics

Minor neuromuscular twitches, tics have been treated successfully at times by the use of hypnosis. Sometimes the tics disappear if they are ignored; at other times, regardless of the therapy, they persist.

Recurrent Aphthous and Herpetic Lesions

Recurrent aphthous and herpetic lesions comprise another group of stress-related conditions that has been treated with a multitude of methods. Some of the methods used include the following: (1) vitamin B injections; (2) application of tetracyclines, gentian violet, silver nitrate, corticosteroids, Orabase® HCA (a protective emollient), peroxide mixes (Gly-Oxide® and Proxigel®); and (3) saline and various other mouthwashes. To reduce the incidence of these lesions, the practice of meditation and self-hypnosis might be helpful.

Miscellaneous Conditions

With respect to the various miscellaneous stress-related conditions, such as metallic taste, gagging, burning tongue, trismis, paresthesia, and atypical facial neuralgia, the use of antianxiety drugs, psychological relaxation techniques, and psychological consultation should prove helpful. Recently, Charles Scialfa (1978) has reported the successful use of the Jankelson Myo-Monitor® (a portable electronic instrument that generates an electrical current) to treat stress-related oral and facial pain and paresthesia.

Summary

All of the treatments for the stress-related oral conditions have two principal aspects. The first is the use of specific methods to overcome the local factors. The second is the use of nonspecific modalities to reduce the effects of psychological stressors. The most effective antistress methods for conditions such as NUG, bruxism, and myofascial pain-dysfunction syndrome are the use of psychological techniques such as meditation, hypnosis, progressive relaxation, autogenic training, and biofeedback.

REFERENCES

Atterbury, R. A.: Auditory pre-sedation for oral surgery patients. *Cal, 38(6)*:2, 1974.

Baldwin, D. C., Jr.: An investigation of psychological and behavioral responses in dental extraction in children. *J Dent Res (Suppl 6), 45*:1637, 1966.

Barber, T. X., Spanos, L. P., and Chaves, J. F.: *Hypnosis, Imagination, and Human Potentialities*. New York, Pergamon, 1974.

Barenie, J. T. and Ripa, L. W.: The use of behavior modification techniques to successfully manage the child dental patient. *JADA, 94*:329, 1977.

Baseheart, J. R.: Nonverbal communication in the dentist-patient relationship. *J Prosthet Dent, 34*:4, 1975.

Beck, F. M.: Placebos in dentistry: Their profound potential effects. *JADA, 95:*1122, 1977.

Benson, H., Beary, J. F., and Carol, M. P.: The Relaxation Response. *Psychiatry, 37:*37, 1974.

Bloomfield, H. H., Cain, M. P., and Jaffe, D. T.: *TM: Discovering Inner Energy and Overcoming Stress.* New York, Delacorte, 1975.

Bloomfield, J.: The initial interview. *Dent Clin North Am, 6:*601, 1962.

Borland, L. R.: Odontophobia — Inordinate fear of dental treatment. *Dent Clin North Am, 6:*683, 1962.

Budyznski, T. and Stoyva, J.: An electromyographic feedback technique for teaching voluntary relaxation of the masseter muscle. *J Dent Res, 52:*116, 1973.

Cannistraci, A. J.: A method to control bruxism: Biofeedback-assisted relaxation therapy. *J Am Soc Prev Dent, 6(12):*12, 1976.

Carlsson, S. G., Gale, E. N., and Öhman, A.: Treatment of temporomandibular joint syndrome with biofeedback training. *JADA, 91:*602, 1975.

Carrel, R. and Binns, W. H., Jr.: The time for office sedation has arrived. *Gen Dent, 25(3):*44, 1977.

Cassidy, J. E.: How to prevent dental phobia. *J Pedo, 1:*21, Fall, 1976.

Christen, A. G.: Improving the child's dental behavior through mental rehearsal. *Northwest Dent, 50:*223, 1972.

Cinotti, W. R., Grieder, A., and Springob, H. K.: *Applied Psychology in Dentistry,* 2nd ed. St. Louis, Mosby, 1972, pp. 94-101.

Clarke, N. G. and Kardachi, B. J.: The treatment of myofascial pain-dysfunction syndrome using the biofeedback principle. *J Periodontol, 48:*643, 1977.

Cosgrove, D.: Sedation in dentistry. *Aust Dent J, 21:*128, 1976.

Dunlap, J. E.: Do you have a waiting room? *Dent Econ, 67(12):*68, 1977.

Editorial: Feeling tense on subway? Leave. *Philadelphia Evening Bulletin,* 10, Nov. 8, 1977.

Editorial: Mysterious headaches may point to bruxism. *Dent Prod Rep,* 48, March, 1976.

Editorial: Tension causes MPD disorders in women. *JADA, 92:*893, 1976.

Editorial: TV helps young patients relax. *Dent Surv, 53(1):*98, 1977.

Eidelman, D.: A psychological aspect of dentistry. *Sven Tandlak Tidskr, 66:*393, 1973.

Evans, F. J.: The placebo response in pain reduction. *Adv Neurol, 4:*289, 1974.

Firestein, S. K.: Patient anxiety and dental practice. *JADA, 93:*1180, 1976.

Gale, E. N. and Ayer, W. A.: .Treatment of dental phobias. *JADA, 73:*1304, 1969.

Gessel, A. H.: Electromyographic biofeedback and tricyclic antidepressants in myofascial pain-dysfunction syndrome: Psychological predictors of outcome. *JADA, 91:*1048, 1975.

Giddon, D. B.: Psychophysiology of the oral cavity. *J Dent Res (Suppl. 6), 45:*1627, 1966.

Goldman, W.: *Marathon Man.* New York, Delacorte, 1974.

Goldstein, I. C. and Dragon, A. I.: Restorative dentistry under general anesthesia for the exceptional child — As an office procedure. *J Dent Child, 34:*395, Sept., 1967.

Greene, C. S. and Laskin, D. M.: Meprobamate therapy for the myofascial pain-dysfunction (MPD) syndrome: A double-blind evaluation. *JADA, 82:*587, 1971.

Hassett, J.: Why dentists are a pain in the mind. *Psychol Today, 11(8):*60, 1978.

Hilgard, E. R., Atkinson, R. C., and Atkinson, R. L.: Techniques of psychotherapy. In Hilgard, E. R. (Ed.): *Introduction to Psychology,* 6th ed. New York, HarBrace J, 1975, pp. 497-521.

Hilgard, E. R. and Hilgard, J. R.: *Hypnosis in the Relief of Pain.* Los Altos, Calif., William Kaufmann, 1975.

Holbroyd, S. V.: *Clinical Pharmacology in Dental Practice.* St. Louis, Mosby, 1974.

Ivanov-Smolensky: *Essays on the Pathophysiology of the Higher Nervous Activity According to Pavlov and his School.* Moscow, Foreign Language Publishing House, 1954.

Jacobson, E.: *Anxiety and Tension Control.* Philadelphia, Lippincott, 1964.

Kleinknecht, R. A., Klepac, R. K., and Alexander, L. D.: Origins and characteristics of fear of dentistry. *JADA, 86:*842, 1973.

Lamb, D. H. and Plant, R.: Patient anxiety in the dentist's office. *J Dent Res, 51:*986, 1972.

Lang, P. J.: Experimental studies of fear reduction. *J Dent Res, 45:*1618, 1966.

Langa, H.: *Relative Analgesia in Dental Practice: Inhalation Analgesia with Nitrous Oxide,* 2nd ed. Philadelphia, Saunders, 1976.

Laskin, D. M. and Greene, C. S.: Influence of the doctor-patient relationship on placebo therapy for patients with myofascial pain-dysfunction (MPD) syndrome. *JADA, 85:*892, 1972.

Lazarus, R. S.: Some principles of psychological stress and their relation to dentistry. *J Dent Res (Suppl. 6), 45:*1620, 1966.

Levoy, R. P.: Do questions from your patients bug you? *Dent Econ, 67(3):*95, 1977.

Lowell, R. J.: Restorative dentistry under general anesthesia. *Oral Surg, 18:*42, 1964.

Luthe, W.: *Autogenic Training.* New York, Grune, 1969.

Melamed, B. G., Weinstein, D., Hawes, R., and Katin-Borland, M.: Reduction of fear-related dental management problems with the use of filmed modeling. *JADA, 90:*822, 1975.

Melzack, R. and Wall, P. D.: Pain mechanisms: A new theory. *Science, 150:*971, 1965.

Messer, J. G.: Stress in dental patients undergoing routine procedures. *J Dent Res, 56:*362, 1977.

Miller, N. E. and Dworkin, B. R.: Effects of learning on visceral functions — Biofeedback. *N Engl J Med, 296:*1274, 1977.

Morse, D. R.: Nitrous oxide analgesia and endodontic practice. *J Natl Anal Soc, 1:*22, 1972.

——: *Clinical Endodontology: A Comprehensive Guide to Diagnosis, Treatment and Prevention.* Springfield, Ill., Thomas, 1974, pp. 379-413.

——: Hypnosis in the practice of endodontics. *J Am Soc Psychosom Dent Med, 22(1):*17, 1975.

——: Use of a meditative state for hypnotic induction in the practice of endodontics. *Oral Surg, 41:*664, 1976.

——: An exploratory study of the use of meditation alone and in combination with hypnosis in clinical dentistry. *J Am Soc Psychosom Dent Med, 24(4):*113, 1977a.

——: Rebuttal to a JAMA editorial. *JADA, 95:*23, 1977b.

——: Variety, exercise, meditation can relieve practice stress. *Dent Stud, 56(3):*26, 1977c.

——: The practice building spell. *Dent Surv, 54(3):*20, 1978.

Morse, D. R. and Hildebrand, C. N.: Case report: Use of TM in periodontal therapy. *Dent Surv, 52(11):*36, 1976.

Morse, D. R., Martin, J. S., Furst, M. L., and Dubin, L. L.: A physiological and subjective evaluation of meditation, hypnosis and relaxation. *Psychosom Med, 39:*304, 1977.

——: *A Physiological and Subjective Evaluation of the Use of Neutral and Emotionally-Charged Words for Meditation.* Abstract No. 695. Abstracts AAAS Annual Meeting, Washington, D.C., 1978.

Pinkham, J. R. and Schroeder, C. S.: Dentist and psychologist: Practical considerations for a team approach to the intensely anxious dental patient. *JADA, 90:*1022, 1975.

Protell, M. R., Krasner, J. D., and Fabrikant, B.: *Psychodynamics in Dental Practice.* Springfield, Ill., Thomas, 1975, pp. 194-218.

Reyes-Guerra, A., Jr.: IV sedation and analgesia — Alternatives to general anesthesia. *Dent Surv, 52(5):*52, 1976.

Rich, P. R.: Music calms the "angry beast" of pain. *Dent Stud, 55(7):*47, 1977.

Rosenberg, J. L.: Psychological evaluation of physical aspects of the dental office. *Dent Clin North Am, 6:*709, 1962.

Schmidt, D. A.: Creating the climate for successful dentistry. *Dent Manag, 17(5):*43, 1977.

Schmidt, D.: Sounds that sell dentistry. *Dent Manag, 18(1):*67, 1978.

Schwartz, W.: Treatment of children. In Protell, M. R., Krasner, J. D., and Fabrikant, B.: *Psychodynamics in Dental Practice.* Springfield, Ill., Thomas, 1975, pp. 159-193.

Scialfa, C. T.: Electrical stimulation for the treatment of facial paresthesia and pain. *Dent Surv, 54(1):*42, 1978.

Ship, I. I.: Epidemiologic aspects of recurrent apthous ulcerations. *Oral Surg, 33:*400, 1972.

Simon, M.: Magic offers key to gaining rapport with young patients. *Dent Surv, 52(12)*:43, 1976.

Simon, W. J.: Proper patient management begins with able assistant. *Dent Surv, 53(2)*:39, 1977.

Travell, J.: Temporomandibular joint pain referred from muscles of the head and neck. *J Prosthet Dent, 10*:745, 1960.

Vaisrub, S.: Hepatitis B — Traffic in the dentist's office. *JAMA, 232*:1270, 1975.

Venham, L. and Quatrocelli, S.: The young child's response to repeated dental procedures. *J Dent Res, 56*:734, 1977.

Vollmer, D.: Your case presentation: Accentuate the positive. *Dent Manag, 16(10)*:79, 1976.

Voss, L. and Shimoda, T.: Protect against free NO_2 in the operatory — For health's sake. *Dent Stud, 55(8)*:62, 1977.

Walrath, L. C. and Hamilton, D. W.: Autonomic correlates of meditation and hypnosis. *Am J Clin Hypn, 17*:190, 1975.

Weisenberg, M. and Epstein, D.: Patient training as an alternative to general anesthesia. *NY Dent J, 39*:610, 1973.

Weiss, J.: Watch your language! Patients do! *Dent Manag, 15(12)*:57, 1975.

Witteman, J. K.: Symposium on Behavioral and Managerial Considerations in Dental Practice. *Dent Clin North Am, 21(3)*, 1977.

Wolpe, J. and Lazarus, A. A.: *Behavior Therapy Techniques.* Oxford, Pergamon, 1966.

Wynne, L.: Synthesis of appropriate patient behavior in an aversive dental environment. *Percept Mot Skills, 38*:519, 1974.

Zeldow, L. L.: Treating clenching and bruxing by habit change. *JADA, 93*:31, 1976.

CHAPTER 6

OVERCOMING DENTIST STRESS

Methods of coping with dentist stress during schooling, practice, teaching, and personal life are covered. Considered are (1) physical and psychological coping methods, including avoidance, denial, and diversion; (2) the relaxation response and sleep; (3) eating and drinking; (4) smoking, drug intake, and inhalation sedation; (5) massage and heat; (6) exercise; (7) laughing and crying; (8) pacing and rocking; (9) talking and whistling; and (10) consultation. The management of stress-related symptoms, diseases, and disorders is examined.

OVERCOMING THE STRESS OF PROFESSIONAL AND PRIVATE LIFE

Introduction

PAUL REVERE was a silversmith and freedom fighter. Zane Grey wrote many popular Western novels. Casey Stengel managed the New York Yankees for many years. Cary Middlecoff was a great golfer, and Billy Cannon helped give the American Football League professional recognition. Gary Cuozzo was a star NFL quarterback. Peter George was an Olympic middleweight weight-lifting champion. Irwin Dambrot was a superb college basketball player. This diversity of endeavors is demonstrated by others who have been congressmen, governors, chancellors of universities, race car drivers, movie makeup men, screen writers, business executives, movie stars, and financial wizards.

What did they all have in common? Each one was a dentist who either combined his dental practice with another career or left the active practice of dentistry for an alternative life-style. Although this is not the only way to cope with the stress of dentistry, it is a key concept which is expressed in the saying,

"Variety is the spice of dentistry!" (Weiss, 1977).

The various ways to cope with the stress of dentistry are now considered. As discussed in Chapter 1, stress may be divided into three major components: the stressors, the individual makeup and the stress response. Stress management involves each of these three components: (1) Stressors can be effectively handled either by avoidance or evasion. One way to avoid stressors is to take a vacation. (2) To better cope with stressors, the individual's makeup should be toughened. Two ways that this may be accomplished are by physical and mental preparation. Physical preparation includes exercise, optimum nutrition, sleep, and rest. Mental preparation includes planning and rehearsal. (3) The stress response can be changed from distress to eustress; two ways of achieving this are through exercise and positive thinking.

An effective method of dealing with stress is to try to compensate for the repetitive episodes of stress by regularly eliciting the response opposite to stress; namely, the relaxation response. The relaxation response can be facilitated by several methods, including meditation, hypnosis, structured relaxation, and napping.

In the remainder of this chapter, the various methods of positive stress management are examined, along with the negative coping methods, e.g. drinking, drugs, and smoking. Stress management is considered under the various phases and types of dental practice.

Dental Personality and Schooling

Coping with the stress of dentistry should begin before one even becomes a dentist. It should start when an individual first considers dentistry as a career. As discussed in Chapter 3, people who engage in a profession they dislike show more evidence of distress than individuals who are in a profession from which they derive satisfaction. Hence, the first consideration is that a person should not enter dentistry unless he believes that he will enjoy it. If he is presently a practicing dentist, he should try to derive some pleasure from the choice of his profession (Borland, 1977). If this is not possible, then he should seriously consider another career or occupation for his health's sake (Box 6-1).

Box 6-1: The Satisfied Dentist

> The strong association between dissatisfaction and distress was supported in a recent study involving Canadian dentists. The investigators found that dentists who derived a high degree of satisfaction from their work showed much less evidence of distress than dentists who were not happy in their occupation (Howard et al., 1976). With respect to this matter, in a fifteen-year longitudinal study, it was found that job and career satisfaction are definitely connected to health and are the best predictors of longevity (Palmore, 1969).

Another consideration for the prospective dentist is the chance for independence that so many dental students rate as the key motivational factor in the choice of dentistry (*see* Chap. 3). Independence in dentistry ordinarily goes hand in hand with lack of professional contact, which can lead to distress. As was the case with job satisfaction, lack of contact can be detrimental to health (Box 6-2).

Box 6-2: The Perils of Isolation

> In a recently concluded nine-year longitudinal study, Lisa Berkman found that people with few strong social relationships had an increased mortality rate as compared to those with many social relationships. The socially isolated were two to four and one-half times more likely to die of any given disease than were their gregarious counterparts (Editorial: Loneliness, 1977).

Thus, it may be that dentists should think twice about that solo practice. Consideration should be given to alternatives such as (1) partnerships, (2) business associations, (3) group practice, and (4) part-time teaching, hospital affiliation, lecturing, consultation, and administration. Dentists should also consider community and organization involvement; they should seek some association with interesting people engaged in activities that fall outside the scope of dentistry.

The solo practice also leads to monotony and fatigue. The beginning dentist should realize that his first office, despite its investment in elaborate equipment and furniture, may not be the only office in his career. He should be prepared to change equipment, furnishings, staff, and even locations to offset the tendency for distress that can result from going to the same office and seeing the same faces year after year.

The individual considering dentistry also should realize that mechanical skills are more important in dentistry than in medicine. Even though dentistry does have the potentialities for teaching, research and administration, mechanical aptitude is still of major importance. To practice nonclinical dentistry, such as in doing research, it is still necessary to satisfactorily complete all clinical requirements while in dental school. Hence, the mechanically limited student has two alternatives. The first is to abandon the thought of being a dentist. The second is to apply to a dental school where mechanical skills are not the crucial requirement, e.g. the Harvard School of Dental Medicine.

A final consideration for the prospective student is financial. The cost of a combined college-dental school education is enormous. This is probably more of a stress factor for the parents than for the student, although the student might have guilt feelings about taking money from his parents. Some students partly compensate for the guilt by working part-time. For the student with low- or middle-income background, there are many scholarships available, and these can help reduce this potentially stressful problem.

The other financial question for the prospective student is, "How much can I make in dentistry?" The would-be dentist should realize that a good living can be made in dentistry, but one ordinarily does not become a millionaire. To avoid future stress, one may have to reset financial sights to a more realistic level.

With the prevailing methods of selection into dental schools, it is difficult to completely avoid the stress that results from competition for grades. Yet, there are certain ways to cope. One way is to plan ahead and develop regular study habits. A second is to realize that failure in one exam or even one course is not the end of a dental career; often, there is a second chance. A third method of coping is to begin early in life to develop potentially healthful patterns, such as regular, vigorous exercise, balanced nutrition, and sufficient rest, relaxation, sleep, and diversion. Adequate rest and relaxation along with regular physical activity often result in a mentally alert student who can study well.

At the present time, dental education imposes stressors on the dental student. Without addressing ourselves to the rationale for the existing dental educational policies, it is believed that there are ways of coping with some of the more trying circumstances. Student participation on curriculum committees can help offset the anxieties induced by the demands of a rigorous dental education. In addition, the requirements of dental education are beginning to reflect student input. For example, basic science courses are becoming more relevant in that there is greater emphasis on applications to dentistry. There is greater emphasis on practice management. Methods of anxiety control, such as nitrous oxide-oxygen analgesia, I.V. sedation, and hypnosis are being offered to undergraduate dental students. And courses and departments of behavioral science are being instituted in many schools to train students in the sociological and psychological aspects of dentistry.

Perhaps written evaluations by students of their teachers can help in improving teaching methods. It may be that changes will come about as a result of discussions between student representatives and school administrators. A concerted effort by students, faculty, administration, and alumni might lead to the introduction of better clinical facilities and updated equipment.

The stress of taking state board examinations cannot be eliminated at this time. However, the advent of regional examinations and reciprocity between states has decreased the number of required examinations. In addition, many states are giving more appropriate tests. For instance, although gold foils may be seen as a measure of high-quality dentistry, these very demanding procedures have been eliminated as a requirement for some board exams. Hence, the future looks brighter.

Dental Practice

In The Beginning

It is difficult to cope with the stresses of the beginning practice. However, the new practitioner can get help. Local community leaders and dental supply salesmen can assist in the selection of an office location. Dental dealers are also helpful in the selection of equipment and supplies. Yet, the starting dentist should not become overcommitted. He should not begin with a large office, e.g. 2,000 square feet of space, and four treatment rooms of equipment. A more modest investment in space and equipment reduces the cost of rent and equipment loans.

Business management is often difficult for the starting dentist. The new dentist is faced with ordering supplies, training and managing staff, regulating the schedule, dealing with the lab, balancing the books, collecting payments, and threats of malpractice. The time to get help is before the practice burgeons. There are many excellent dental business management firms. The monetary investment is well worth the price to insure future security and decreased stress levels. Periodic staff meetings with the opportunity for feedback are essential. It is also important to get a good accountant, lawyer, and financial advisor. The dentist should not get overly involved with investments and insurances beyond his means. In order to invest and sufficiently insure oneself, it is mandatory that sound professional advice be sought. Having adequate fire, malpractice, disability, and life insurance can help with the many stressful events that may occur.

To help prevent malpractice suits, dentists should —

1. Have patients fill out and sign medical and dental questionnaires;

2. Not attempt cases beyond their expertise;
3. Make definitive financial arrangements with each patient;
4. Take adequate x-rays, photographs, study models, and other diagnostic tests throughout the treatment;
5. Keep complete records for each patient;
6. Try to maintain rapport with each patient, but they should not be overly friendly;
7. Inform patients in advance about possible untoward occurrences, e.g. the possibility of apicoectomy causing paresthesia;
8. Explain problems to patients and refer the patients to recognized specialists, e.g. broken root canal instrument — refer the case to an endodontist;
9. Be wary of accepting patients who are "shoppers";
10. Be cautious about suing patients for small overdue accounts; malpractice suits often result; and
11. Consider countersuing patients if they feel the suits are unwarranted.

The fledgling dentist should not be depressed if he doesn't reach his financial goal after the first year. All too often, he becomes depressed (Box 6-3). The beginning dentist should consider the adage "Rome wasn't built in a day." Judging from prior years of experience, the first year is not an accurate barometer of the future of a dental practice. After a few years, most dentists are able to pay back their outstanding loans and still achieve some financial independence.

The stress produced by the association with an established practitioner is difficult to avoid. It is most important to obtain a trial period of at least six months in order to help determine whether or not a more permanent relationship is feasible.

Box 6-3: Money Woes For The New Dentist

The depression-prone new dentist was highlighted in the recent *Dental Management* survey of the graduating class of 1976 at the University of Texas at Houston. After one year of practice, many of the 1976 graduates had financial problems and reported being depressed with their money plight (Green, 1977).

Ideal versus Practical

To prevent disconcerting stress reactions, the new dentist has to be able to separate the ideal dentistry that he was taught in dental school from the real world of practical dentistry. This does not mean he should perform shoddy dentistry, as that can also be stressful. But he must realize the following:

1. Salesmanship is part of dentistry.

2. People paying off home mortgages and car loans do not always give comprehensive dentistry a high priority.

3. Dental patients are not manikins. Not only are there lips, a tongue, saliva, and vocal cords to contend with, but there is usually more fear and greater expectations with a private patient, as compared to a dental school clinic patient. As discussed in the previous chapter, patients' fears and negative dental images can be overcome. Working in a relaxed environment with tranquil patients is conducive to better dentistry and healthier dentists.

4. Failures can and do occur, and faulty workmanship and uncooperative patients are unavoidable at times. Rigid criteria for success may by themselves be stress inducing. For example, by firm standards, an original periapical area should completely disappear for complete success. Yet, many areas do not disappear entirely, and the case is considered to be a clinical success.

5. There is no shame involved in referring difficult cases to specialists.

6. Specialists should be used for consultations and advice; a specialist does not think less of a generalist who asks for his opinion.

7. The techniques taught in dental school are not immutable. Some schools teach a preferred method that may not be practical or effective in all circumstances or when undertaken by a particular dentist. Dentists may learn better techniques from colleagues at continuing-education courses.

8. Local anesthesia is not always 100 percent effective. If pain occurs either during treatment or between visits, the

dentist should do his best to resolve the problem, e.g. give an intrapulpal injection or prescribe narcotics. However, if the practitioner did his best, he should not blame himself for the patient's pain. Often, the pain occurs because of the patient's neglect.

9. Treating the patient is the responsibility of the dentist, but the dentist does have a life of his own. He should not be married to his practice. As long as the patients are not abandoned, the dentist should feel free to decrease his stress level by taking frequent vacations and participating in nondental activities, e.g. hobbies, athletics, reading, going to shows, meetings, theaters, sporting events, and dining out. Wherever the new dentist practices, there are generally other competent dentists around. There should be cooperation between practitioners, so each can cover the other's emergencies. In time, associates may enter the practice, and then cooperation can be assured. An important point for the dentist working alone is this: He should not worry about losing his patients to other dentists if he is not always present. Patients generally are more loyal than dentists give them credit to be. If dentists lose their patients regularly, then it is time for them to reevaluate both their technical methods and personal interrelationships.

The Positive Service

The dentist should realize and let his patients know that he is performing a positive psychological as well as mechanical service. As discussed in Chapter 2, the oral cavity has profound psychological significance. Therefore, for those patients who may fear dental intervention, saving teeth can preclude patients' fears of aging, mutilation, and the (Freudian) fear of castration.

A long-lasting toothache can make an individual irritable, excitable, unfriendly, and depressed. Alleviation of the pain by endodontic therapy or extraction can restore the individual to a more positive mental state. Patients may also have severe bouts of depression because of ugly teeth and malocclusions. Restoring their mouths to a normal appearance can often change the individuals' outlooks on life. In the case where a patient's tooth was previously mobile and mastication of many foods was difficult, the result of having a firm tooth (possibly by the use of a periodontal splint, an endodontic implant, or a fixed bridge) may permit the patient to eat foods previously avoided. The significant consequence may be a happier individual who can enjoy his meals more.

The dentist's realization that he is improving the psychological health of his patients can enhance his own self-image. But for the sake of his own sanity, the dentist should not be a psychologist or psychiatrist to his patients. He should have empathy but should not take the patient's problems for his own. He should remain friendly but firm, which is in keeping with the role of the competent professional.

The Mechanics of Dentistry

To overcome the problems caused by the physical proximity of the patient and dentist, the dentist should —

1. Wear a mask to prevent the inhalation of infectious viruses and microbes, e.g. hepatitis; noxious gases; toxic chemicals; foul odors from putrescent root canals; and patients' bad breath.
2. Not hover over the patient. Working by indirect vision can help maintain the patient and dentist at a comfortable working distance that would not interfere with the patient's personal space.
3. Alternate between standing and sitting to allow for both rest and exercise.
4. Refrain from bending to prevent back problems.

To overcome the problems caused by monotony and fatigue, the dentist should alternate various procedures (and possibly even working hours) during the day. For example, a difficult surgery case might be followed by a simple restorative procedure. The office hours might begin at 9 AM one day and 1 PM the following day.

Teaching

The stress of dental teaching was discussed in Chapter 3. Now let us consider some of the positive rewards of teaching. These include (1) the opportunity to engage in research that can improve the practice of dentistry; (2) being able to keep up with the dental literature; (3) being able to observe the most recent techniques; (4) the opportunity to instruct well-motivated students; (5) the chance for friendship, companionship, sharing of ideas, and discussion of cases; (6) the opportunity to write and lecture in continuing-education courses; (7) the opportunity to attend outside courses or give courses while still being compensated (varies with the school); (8) fringe benefits, e.g. health and life insurances and tuition remission; and (9) security (once tenure is obtained).

On balance, the positive aspects of teaching may outweigh the negative stress-inducing factors. Still, one must consider the personal pros and cons to teaching before giving up private practice. Many potential stress-inducing situations can be avoided if there is forethought given (Morse, 1978).

Goals

One way to prevent distress is to set realistic goals. The dentist should carefully choose his career goals and should not be afraid to make a change if the situation becomes unbearable (Box 6-4). In reference to goals, it should be realized that it takes time to reach objectives. Impatience engenders stress. Hence, the dentist should plan carefully and exercise patience.

Box 6-4: The Chameleon Authors

The sequence of careers enjoyed by the senior author (D.M.) is as follows: microbiologist, teacher, general practitioner, and endodontist; and for the junior author (M.F.): aerospace engineer, business executive (electronics industry), teacher, and psychologist. Even though there was stress involved in the several career changes or additions, both individuals report that, overall, positive results were experienced.

A Sound Mind in a Sound Body

Introduction

Whether one is in practice or teaching and follows the suggestions given above, there are still petty day-to-day conflicts and aggravations. It is important that the dentist realizes when these problems are becoming serious. He should become sensitive to signs of stress, such as chronic anxiety, depression, and hostility. These indicate that all is not well. The dentist should search for the sources of the hidden frustrations or conflicts and then do something constructive about them. Even more important than treatment is prevention. Sometimes a condition such as ulcers may not respond to medication. Hence, complete avoidance of the stress-inducing situation might be indicated.

There are a number of ways to achieve positive results. Unfortunately, some of the methods have deleterious side effects. The various methods of prevention and coping with distress are now discussed.

Avoidance

The first way to prevent distress is to physically avoid as many possible stressful situations as one can. For instance, if the dentist cannot manage children, then he should refer his child patients to a pedodontist.

Evasion

When a stressful situation cannot be avoided, sometimes it may be sidestepped. For example, in an emotionally charged situation where a vote for either side may elicit stress, one could abstain. However, evasion itself may be stressful. Hence, this way out should be used sparingly.

Effective Action

If the dentist faces a new situation that goes against old habits of thought and action, he is much more likely to become severely stressed than if he faces a stressful situation that he has met before. In order to best handle a new situation, one should be mentally and physically prepared (Fig. 6-1). This entails planning or rehearsal. For example, if as result of many rehearsals a dentist is well prepared to handle a medical emergency, then he would be less apt to go into shock himself in the event a patient had a cardiac seizure in the dental chair.

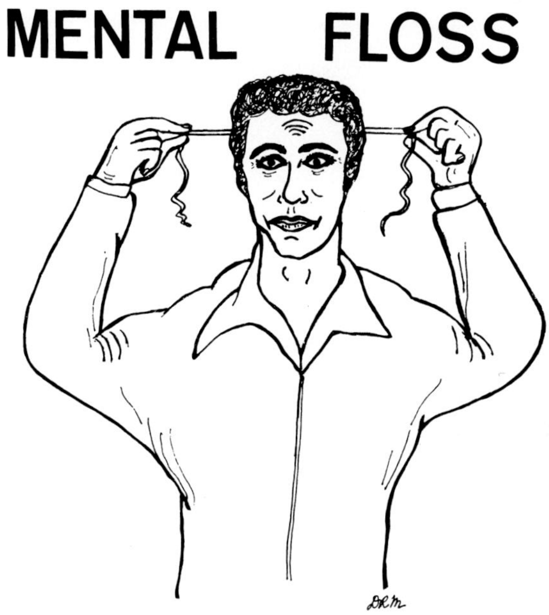

Figure 6-1. Just as dental flossing is important in coping with dental caries, so is "mental flossing" (mental preparation) important in coping with stressors.

Insulation

If a dentist knows from previous experience that a particular situation will be stressful and he cannot avoid the situation, then the best response is often no response. For instance, if a particular individual is loud and vehement in his personal attacks, rather than counterattacking, it might be preferable to say yes to him and thus avoid greater stress.

A Kind Word

With reference to the "loud" individual, sometimes a smile or a few pleasant words might change a potentially distressing situation into one that yields eustress. Hence, a dentist should try to replace anger with joy, negative criticism with praise, and fear with relaxation.

Mental Repetition

Dentists should not dwell on misfortunes. The cliché about not crying over spilled milk is appropriate. Rehashing the past only increases psychological stressors, such as frustration, anger, and anxiety (Box 6-5).

Box 6-5: Mental Tennis

> Timothy Gallwey in his book, *The Inner Game of Tennis* (1974), has illustrated vividly the perils of living in the past. Many fewer errors are made when one concentrates on his breathing or on seeing the ball, i.e. a form of meditation, than when a mental replay is made of the previous point.

Defensive Mechanisms

The previously mentioned coping mechanisms, such as avoidance, evasion, effective action, and insulation, involve flexibility and choice. Conversely, defense mechanisms such as denial, rationalization, and regression involve behavior that is rigid and automatized. In general, the more intense the response is to stress, the greater the use of defense mechanisms to reduce the emotional hurt and to justify the ways in which one responds.

If the situation is unbearable and there is danger of upset to the mental equilibrium, then rationalization or denial might be helpful temporarily. However, this line of defense should not be held at all costs. For instance, denying the possibility of cancer when a growth in the mouth is present in order to avoid a trip to the dentist, might lead to death.

Rationalization might help maintain sanity for the moment. Two typical examples come to mind: (1) A dentist boasts of his fabulous income and of all the great places to which he has been. He may be engaging in this behavior as a cover for his boring practice that he hates. (2) If a dentist did not like doing amalgams all day, he might rationalize that he was performing an indispensable service. Of course, the service has real value, but in this case, it is given at the expense of the dentist. It should be realized that the prolonged use of defensive mechanisms to cope with stress can cripple a person psychologically and physically and may lead to severe neuroses and psychoses.

Diversion

A dentist's professional life contains many day-to-day chronic stressors, and it is important to break away from the routine. Hobbies, reading, entertainment, and vacations are all important (Box 6-6). But when that trip is taken or that artistic masterpiece is created, the dentist should not mentally take the dental practice along with him. The dentist should change his internal orientation to an external focus. Continually mulling over problems generally intensifies them, and worry is counterproductive. Getting out of the immediate environment and seeking others may give a healthy distance to the problems.

During vacations, it is important that the dentist get rest as well as exercise. But the dentist should not program his vacation as he programs his practice. The vacation should be free-floating. Dentists should not consider vacations merely as an escape from a demanding or boring practice. Apparently, many dentists tend to look toward their next vacation as soon as they finish the first. This should not be the case. While the immediate object may be to remove himself from the dental setting, the vacation should restore the dentist's capability to undertake the workload once again.

Box 6-6: A Lesson To Be Learned From TV Addiction

Watching TV is a daily diversion of many people. Although there may be fine shows on televison, there is also inanity, sex, and violence. Possible physical damage includes eyestrain, hearing loss, and radiation effects, i.e. from sitting too close to color TV. Passive TV watching also affords less opportunity for interaction between people and can limit constructive work and exercise.

The *Detroit Free Press* reports that TV viewing can also be quite addicting. Representatives of the newspaper approached 120 families and offered to pay them $500 per family if they would agree not to watch any television for one month. Incredibly, 93 of the 120 families did not accept. Of the 27 families who accepted the offer, 5 had their TV sets temporarily disconnected. They also had problems: One man spent almost the entire month reading newspapers. Two people became chain-smokers. Children in some of the families became cranky and continually begged to have their sets turned back on. But it was not all bad. Some of the families reported that the experience brought them closer together. People also read more, visited other families, and took more vacations (Bricklin, 1978).

Remember that the daily practice must also be rewarding. If it is not, then steps should be taken to alter the situation. For example, one could take courses, read the dental literature, find associates, change working hours, change setups, write articles, or give lectures. If a dentist finds that his practice no longer interests him, he might consider going back to school for specialty training, or he might consider full-time teaching. In fact, if dentistry is no longer exciting, then the discontented dentist might follow in Casey Stengel's footsteps and become a big league manager (or consider another more appropriate career).

Relaxation Response

Each dentist should set aside one or two daily periods of

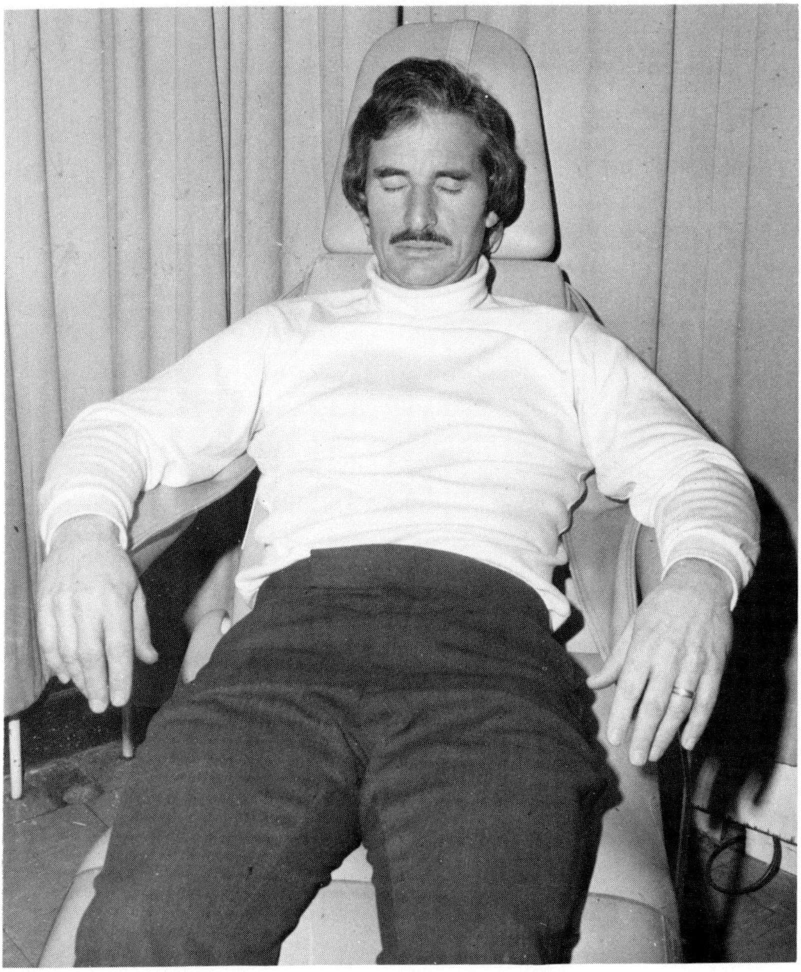

Figure 6-2. The senior author is shown using the combined meditation-hypnosis technique. (From D. R. Morse, Overcoming "Practice Stress" Via Meditation and Hypnosis, *Dental Survey, 53(7)*:32, 1977. Courtesy of *Dental Survey* and Harcourt Brace Jovanovich, Inc., New York, New York.)

twenty to thirty minutes each to practice the relaxation response. Any of the techniques described in Chapter 5 can be effective; some individuals benefit from daydreaming, some meditate, some use a form of self-hypnosis, some use biofeedback-assisted relaxation, others use the combined technique of hypnosis-meditation (Fig. 6-2), and still others combine religion with meditation through daily religious worship. But whatever the method used, it has been found that regular elicitation of the relaxation response is beneficial as a method of coping with stress.

Patricia Carrington (1977, 1978) has devised an interesting method of minimeditations in which short periods of meditation (one to two minutes) coincide with relatively stressful periods of the day. This innovation might refine and enlarge the effects of the two daily longer periods of meditation.

Sleep

Everyone believes that getting enough sleep is essential for good health. Even though eight hours per night is considered normal by most people, just what is enough has not been established scientifically. A recent study, however, has helped in the clarification of "normal" sleep (Box 6-7).

Box 6-7: Salubrious Sleep

A recent longitudinal study by Nedra Belloc (1973) of 7,000 adults sheds some light on the question of what constitutes an adequate amount of sleep. In this study, seven personal health-related practices were measured and correlated with mortality rates. The seven practices were as follows: (1) sleeping habits, (2) eating or missing breakfast, (3) snacking or not snacking between meals, (4) maintenance of "normal" body weight, (5) regularity of exercise, (6) frequency of drinking alcoholic beverages, and (7) smoking habits.

With respect to sleep, it was found that people who slept eight hours nightly had a lower mortality rate than those who slept seven hours nightly. The eight-hour sleepers had a 50 percent lower mortality rate than people who slept six hours or less. Interestingly enough, those who slept nine hours or more nightly also had an increased mortality rate, in comparison with the eight-hour sleepers. (They may have slept longer because of illness.)

Eating and Drinking

Aside from the nutritional significance and the pleasures derived, eating is also a means of coping with stressors. Unfortunately, detrimental weight gain is associated with compulsive eating. What and how people eat can affect the ability to cope with the many stressors of life (Box 6-8). For some "fat" people, their layer of fat seems to act as an insulation to the "cruel outer world."

Box 6-8: Gravedigging With One's Teeth

With reference to Belloc's study (1973) involving the seven health-related practices, it was found that eating habits are important. The subjects who ate breakfast almost every day had significantly lower mortality rate than those who consistently missed breakfasts. On the other hand, snacking between meals was associated with a higher mortality. With respect to those of "normal" weight, i.e. those subjects who kept their weight within average weight-height adjusted limits, it was found that they had the lowest mortality rates.

As discussed in Chapter 4, four of the major risk factors for coronary disease are related to eating. To reiterate, those risk factors are (1) elevated serum cholesterol and triglycerides, (2) high salt intake, (3) high carbohydrate intake, and (4) obesity.

In terms of coping with stressors, are there advantages or disadvantages in chewing, eating, or drinking certain foods, beverages, or nutritional supplements? There are some important points to consider. First, there are some food additives, such as artificial colors, flavors, preservatives, stabilizers, and emulsifiers, that are potentially carcinogenic agents. Hence, these definitely should be considered to be acting as stressors.

Next, a common way of coping with stressors is to chew such things as gum or tobacco. Unfortunately, the chewing tobacco or sucrose-containing gum presents health problems. Tobacco contains nicotine, and while sugarless gum containing xylitol may prevent caries, the drug has been implicated as a carcinogen. In other words, chewing by itself may be an acceptable method of stress release, but taking into account the substances chewed, even chewing is not completely safe.

Many people drink coffee, tea, and cocoa during work breaks. Unfortunately, drinking caffeinated beverages can also cause distress responses. Caffeine is found in coffee, tea, and cola drinks; theophylline is found in tea; and theobromine is found in cocoa. Collectively, these alkaloids are known as *xanthines.* Caffeine is the most active of the central nervous system stimulants. Xanthines' actions include (1) diuretic action on the kidney; (2) stimulation of the heart muscle (speeds up heart rate and force of contraction); (3) increase of blood pressure and relaxation of smooth muscle, e.g. bronchial muscles; and (4) increase in the secretion of gastric HCl. In short, cumulative results of these xanthine actions can lead to serious disease in susceptible individuals (Box 6-9).

Box 6-9: Coffee's Harmful Effects

One study of 11,000 males by Ralph Paffenbarger and his co-workers showed that the risk of getting peptic ulcers was 1.4 times greater for moderate drinkers of coffee (one or two cups daily) as compared to abstainers. Two studies by Philip Cole of Harvard showed that bladder cancer incidence was related to coffee drinking. In one of the studies, women who drank one or more cups of coffee daily had 2.5 times the risk of developing bladder cancer as did nondrinkers. Studies by Jick and Slone at Boston University on over 12,500 patients showed that "the risks of infarction among those drinking one to five, and six or more cups of coffee per day are estimated to be increased by 60% and 120% respectively" (Boston Collaborative, 1972). Hence, there appears to be a statistical link between coffee drinking and coronary disease.

Excessive drinking of caffeinated beverages can lead to caffeinism. Symptoms include irritability, restlessness, insomnia, headache, and muscle twitches. Classical anxiety states are simulated by individuals who manifest such symptoms. Neuromuscular coordination is also impaired and can lead to poor response to stressors (Manber, 1976).

Drinking warm nonstimulating beverages such as Postum®, herbal teas, milk, and chicken soup may have a relaxing effect and could prove beneficial. Drinking alcoholic beverages is also a means of coping with stressors. A glass of wine (with relatively low alcohol content) may make an individual less responsive, and this could be an asset in a stressful situation. However, getting drunk to the point of stupefaction is definitely not a way to handle stressors, as excessive drinking is also damaging to health (Box 6-10).

Box 6-10: The Dangers of Drink

In Belloc's study (1973) involving health-related practices, a similar mortality rate was found for teetotalers and for those people who drank no more than one or two alcoholic drinks daily. However, alcoholics had a mortality rate two to three times greater than abstainers.

Although the evidence is not overwhelming, it does appear that optimum levels of vitamins, minerals, proteins, and fiber are necessary to adequately cope with stressors. There is controversy over what is an optimal level and under what conditions. One vitamin that appears to be of importance to effectively cope with stressors is vitamin C (Box 6-11).

Box 6-11: The Saga of Vitamin C and a Prisoner's Perilous Plight

Robert Hodges and his co-workers ran an interesting experiment with six prisoners. The prisoners were deprived of vitamin C and then were given varying doses of the vitamin, including a small amount of radioactively tagged vitamin C. By measuring the amount of radioactivity present in the urine, the investigators determined that each prisoner used approximately 3 percent of the existing body pool of vitamin C, regardless of the dose given.

On the fifty-fourth day of study, two of the prisoners escaped. The cell mate of the escaped two was repeatedly interrogated and he finally "admitted full knowledge of the escape and he 'told all' to the authorities." The other prisoners threatened to kill him, and for the next two-week period, he suffered considerable distress. The "squealer" could hardly sleep; he looked pale; he was apprehensive and tremulous. After a two-week period, the warden informed the distraught and agitated prisoner that for his cooperation he would be pardoned as soon as the experiment was over. Immediately afterwards, the prisoner quieted down and became calm and relaxed.

During all this time, the testing had continued. It was found that for the two-week stress period, the prisoner's utilization of vitamin C increased almost threefold. After the two-week period, it returned to the normal baseline. Thus, from the fortuitous results of this study, one may draw the conclusion that vitamin C is needed in higher doses during periods of stress. This possibility has been somewhat confirmed in studies that show that the adrenal glands contain a high content of vitamin C and that stimulation of the adrenal cortex by ACTH causes a rapid depletion of the vitamin C content (Hodges, 1970).

A dose of 500 mg vitamin C daily for the day before and a few days after is suggested for potentially stressful situations, such as surgery. The preferred form is in a time-release capsule to prevent development of crystalluria (kidney stones).*

The vitamin B complex apparently is important in the body's ability to produce an effective stress response. Pantothenic acid (pantothenate) is a major antistress vitamin (Box 6-12).

Box 6-12: Surviving With Pantothenate

Jeffrey Bland discussed in a recent issue of *Pharmacy West*

*A typical preparation is Cevi-Bid (Geriatric Pharmaceutical Corp.)

the role of the various B complex vitamins in stress (Feltman, 1976). Of special importance was pantothenate. Pantothenate is considered to be essential for the proper functioning of the adrenal glands. It is converted to coenzyme A (CoA) in the body. CoA activates the adrenal hormones.

There have been a few animal studies attesting to the role of pantothenate in stress. In one study, rats who were pre-fed with pantothenate swam an average of sixty-two minutes in cold water, while pantothenate-deficient rats swam an average of sixteen minutes. Another study by Roger Williams (1971) was done with two groups of mice. Both groups (A and B) were fed identical diets except that group A had a pantothenate supplement. Group B lived an average of 550 days, while group A mice lived an average of 653 days. In a third study, Szorady (1963) exposed two groups of fifty mice each to total body x-radiation. Group A was pretreated for one week with pantothenate. Group B had no pretreatment. The results showed that mice in group A had a 200 percent longer survival time than group B mice.

Deficiencies of vitamin B_6 (pyridoxine) may trigger neurological irregularities, such as tics, tremors, and twitches. A major deficiency of vitamin B_3 (niacin) can lead to pellagra, which is characterized by severe depression. Vitamin B_1 (thiamine) deficiency, in early stages, often results in fatigue and complaints of lack of energy. Vitamin E also may be important in the stress response (Box 6-13).

Box 6-13: Vitamin E Helps Rats Cope with Stress

There have been a few animal studies involving vitamin E and various stressors. In one study, three groups of rats were fed varying levels of vitamin E over a period of eight weeks. Then they were exposed to high concentrations of ozone. Significantly greater lung damage was found in the low vitamin E-supplemented rats, as compared to the high vitamin E-supplemented rats.

In a second study, two groups of rats were placed in a maze. Whereas all the rats were continually blocked in their attempts to get food, group A received 100 I.U. of vitamin E daily per rat, and group B had no such supplement. After eight days of frustration, the rats were sacrificed and examined for gastric ulcers. It was found that the vitamin E-supplemented rats had significantly fewer ulcers (Feltman, 1976).

In his discussion of vitamins and stress, Bland (Feltman, 1976) reported that vitamin A and vitamin D also are important in resisting stress. Since vitamin D is needed for bony repair, supplementation might be necessary following dental surgery. Vitamin A is needed for soft tissue repair (epithelialization) but also may have another role in stress (Box 6-14).

Box 6-14: Vitamin A Helps Mice Cope and Reduces Ulcers in Humans

Vitamin A has been shown by Eli Seifter (1976) to block some host responses (in mice) for stressors or cortisone administrations. He specifically showed that when mice were given a sarcoma virus along with physical stressors, they had more severe and a greater number of tumors than when they were only given the virus. However, when they were pretreated with vitamin A and then given the sarcoma virus and physical stressors, the mice had a significantly lower incidence and severity of tumors.

It has been reported that twice-a-day administration of vitamin A (50 to 100,000 I.U.) to burn patients reduces gastrointestinal ulcers. The vitamin A-supplemented patients had less than one-third the incidence of ulcers, as compared to a similar group of burn patients who did not receive the vitamin supplementation (Chernov et al., 1971).

Deficiencies of some minerals can also affect the stress response. Magnesium deficiency causes changes in nerve conduction and muscular contractions and has been reported to elicit subjective responses, such as "nervousness" and irritability (Kinderlehrer, 1973). Zinc is important in the repair of wounds, and calcium is crucial for nerve conduction and muscle contraction. Trace elements such as iron, potassium, and iodine are also necessary for an effectual stress response (Bosco, 1978; Morse, 1974).

As with vitamin C, there probably should be higher doses of the vitamin B complex; vitamins E, A, and D; and supplements of minerals during periods of anticipated stress, such as surgery.*

An adequate intake of proteins (for repair of injuries and replacement of cells) and carbohydrates (for energy) is undoubtedly needed during stress. It is advisable to supplement these nutrients, especially during or following surgery.†

There is also evidence that fiber plays a role in stress. Sandford Siegal has documented the role of fiber as a protection against stress-induced peptic ulcers (Box 6-15). High-fiber foods include bran, unrefined grains, cabbage, and other raw vegetables.

Box 6-15: Fiber Ties Up Ulcers

During World War II, American prisoners of war in Japanese prison camps were given a good supplement of rice polishings, which had a high fiber content (derived from the rice kernel). Out of a total of 13,000 prisoners in three camps, only one case of ulcers was reported for the year. When the prisoners were moved out of Japan, the rice-polishings supplement was discontinued, and ulcers became rampant. Conversely, American prisoners who were kept in Hong Kong had an unsupplemented diet and had a high incidence of ulcers. When they were transferred to Japan, their new diets included unmilled grains and bran supplements. The rate of ulcers then rapidly decreased until it approached zero (Siegal, 1975).

---

*Typical preparations are B-C-Bid (Geriatric Pharmaceutical Corp.); Allbee® with C (A. H. Robins); Z-BEC® (A. H. Robins); and Alpha-E® (Barth Vitamin Corp.). Vitamins A and D are found in supplemented milk and cod-liver oil.

†Typical vitamin-mineral food supplements are Carnation Instant Breakfast®, Nutrament®, Instant Nutrament®, and Meritene®.

Drug Intake

In the discussion on eating and drinking, two kinds of drugs were considered in beverages: (1) xanthines and (2) alcohol. There are other drugs that are used to cope with stressors. The review begins with nicotine and smoking.

1. SMOKING: Aside from the pleasure derived from smoking, it is a habitual method of coping with stressors. There is no doubt that smoking is detrimental to health. Heavy cigarette smoking is one of the important risk factors for coronary disease; there is firm evidence of the strong association between smoking and lung cancer. There are other diseases, such as emphysema, in which heavy smoking is implicated (Box 6-16).

Box 6-16: Puffing Life Away

In Belloc's study (1973) involving health-related practices, smokers had a mortality rate double that of nonsmokers. Heavy smokers who quit had a 50 percent higher mortality rate than nonsmokers. With reference to quitting, dentists have cut down on their smoking habits in the last few years. According to the *Survey of Health Professionals: Smoking and Health, 1975* (National Clearing House, 1975), in 1967 to 1969, 34 percent of dentists smoked, as contrasted to 1975, when 23 percent of dentists smoked.

Smoking has also been reported to lessen the ability to cope with stressors. This is related to the finding that smoking decreases the body's stores of vitamin C (Bourquin and Masmanno, 1953).

2. MARIJUANA SMOKING: Marijuana smoking is also used partly for stress release. Apparently there is some health risk in this practice, but the evidence is not as definitive as it is for cigarette smoking.

3. SEDATIVES AND ANTIANXIETY AGENTS: Since dentists have easy accessibility to sedatives and antianxiety agents, it is also easy for them to get hooked on these drugs. However, it would be far more beneficial to their health if dentists used psycholog-

ical relaxation techniques. Nevertheless, there are definitely stressful occasions when the use of a drug such as Valium is indicated. For severe depression, a dentist should seek psychological or psychiatric aid. Psychiatric treatment may include the use of antidepressant drugs, such as lithium carbonate.

4. INHALATION SEDATION: Nitrous oxide-oxygen is an effective sedation for patients. Some dentists and their aides also use nitrous oxide for their own relaxation purposes. An occasional inhalation is not harmful, but chronic use can result in habituation and toxic effects. When a dentist and assistant engage in after-hours nitrous whiffing, a volatile situation is in progress. In addition, there have been reports of accidental deaths and suicides with nitrous oxide as the agent.

5. DRUGS AS SUBSTITUTES FOR AVOIDANCE: In the beginning of this section, the coping method of avoidance of stressors was discussed. Yet, all too often people do not avoid food or drink stressors because they know that if problems occur, they can depend upon a "magic pill" to restore the body's equilibrium. For instance, if someone gets into a terrible argument and develops a headache, he takes an aspirin rather than avoiding the argument in the first place. If he eats hot Mexican food and gets a stomachache, he takes an antacid to counteract the bad effects, rather than avoiding the spicy food.

Unfortunately, all drugs have side effects. It is more logical and healthful to avoid known stressors than to depend upon pills to try to restore nature's balance.

Massage

Most people enjoy a massage and find it to be relaxing. Massage encompasses Swedish massage, use of hand-held vibrators, hydromassage (water under pressure), shower massage (The Shower Massage, by Water Pic®), massage built into contoured chairs (Contour®, by Contour Chair Lounge, Inc.), and rolfing (a dramatic form of deep massage developed by Ida Rolf). One recommended method that may or may not be relaxing is massage by a member of the opposite sex.

Heat

A warm bath, a steam bath, and a sauna are refreshing and relaxing. It is also believed that use of the steam bath and sauna has health value. It is presumed that the heat generated causes loss of excess salts, toxins, and metabolic products (Foley, 1977). However, there is some danger from the high temperatures involved. Too long a period of exposure to the heat can cause fainting and is dangerous to patients with cardiac conditions. A good and effective combination of moderate heat and gentle massage is found in the Jacuzzi whirlpool bath.

*Exercise**

Exercise is paradoxically both a physical stressor and one of the best methods for coping with stressors. It is modern man's way of indulging in the beneficial fight-or-flight response. Not only is there an advantageous release as the result of the muscular work, but exercise itself increases the body's capacity to cope with stressors. However, sudden severe exertion for the out-of-shape individual can result in a life-threatening stress response. Still, the evidence is mounting that regular, strenuous exercise is a major factor in decreasing the incidence of serious diseases and in prolonging life (Box 6-17).

Box 6-17: Run For Your Life

In Nedra Belloc's study (1973) that has been considered throughout this section, it was shown that exercise is a major factor in longevity. It was found that men who often engaged in active sports, e.g. swimming and jogging, had the lowest mortality of all the subjects. The rate was even lower than that of people who never smoked and also did not exercise. Subjects who exercised infrequently had twice the mortality rate of the active exercisers, regardless of their age. Women who exercised had a much lower mortality rate than those women who never exercised.

*The authors wrote this section with the aid of Mr. Jed Margolis and Mrs. Diane Morse, physical education teachers, Cherry Hill, New Jersey.

At the 1977 Annual Meeting of the American Heart Association, Ralph Paffenbarger reported on a study of Harvard University graduates. In the early 1960s, he sent questionnaires to approximately 36,000 alumni. Included were questions about types of sports engaged in, frequency of participation, and incidence of other strenuous activities, e.g. climbing stairs. About half of the alumni responded. In 1972, these alumni or their survivors received a second questionnaire. An analysis of the returns showed that 572 alumni suffered heart attacks, of which 257 had been fatal.

With respect to exercise, it was found that those who exercised casually (burning fewer than 2,000 calories per week) had a 64 percent higher risk of coronary disease than those who exercised regularly and vigorously. The strenuousness of exercise was a much more important factor than risk factors such as smoking, obesity, hypertension, or family history of cardiac diseases. Activities found to be especially effective were swimming, running, handball, squash, and basketball — if played for an hour or more per day. As far as tennis is concerned (the authors' favorite sport), Paffenberger stated that a good, stiff competitive game of singles should be considered strenuous and effective.

Paffenberger also reported on another study, a twenty-two-year survey of longshoremen. Results showed that longshoremen who engaged in heavy, strenuous work suffered only half as many fatal heart attacks, as compared to the longshoremen performing light activities (Editorial: Medicine: Coronary Curb, 1977).

Studies of the Masai warriors again showed the importance of exercise. The Masai exercise regularly and are free of clinical coronary heart disease. Even in cases where atherosclerosis was present, exercise produced an enlargement of the coronary blood vessels such that nutrient and gaseous exchange increased (Mann, 1977).

Keys's study (1970) of coronary heart disease involved individuals engaged in different occupations in seven countries (including Finland, Italy, and the United States). In each of these countries, those individuals engaged in strenuous work had the lowest incidence of coronary heart disease.

While the use of exercise as a means of preventing cardiovascular disease is fairly well established, the evidence for prevention of other diseases is scanty. Two recent animal studies show that exercise may help in the prevention of cancer (Box 6-18).

Box 6-18: Wheeling Away Cancer

> Two recent mice studies were performed in Japan. In the first study, there were three groups of mice: Group A had free access to an exercise wheel in each cage; group B members did not have access to an exercise wheel; and group C had access to an exercise wheel, but the mice were kept in colonies of five. Upon sacrifice, the results showed: (1) group B (low exercise) had a 60 percent incidence of cancerous livers; (2) group C (moderate exercise) had a 35 percent incidence of cancerous livers; and (3) group A (high exercise) had a 23.5 percent cancer incidence.
>
> In a second study by the same investigators, two groups of mice were given the cancer-inducing chemical benzidine. Results showed that the low-exercise mice had a 93 percent incidence of cancer, as compared to the high-exercise mice, who had a 63 percent cancer incidence (Bricklin, 1977).

The way that strenuous exercise helps in coping with stress and preventing coronary disease is related to the following physiological and subjective responses of exercise:

1. Decrease in serum cholesterol and triglycerides
2. Reduction in blood pressure
3. Decrease in heart rate
4. Increase in stroke volume of heart (blood output per heart beat)
5. Increase in oxygen intake
6. Improvement in strength of skeletal, smooth, and cardiac muscles
7. Increase in muscle tone
8. Increase in muscle flexibility
9. Increase in physical endurance (stamina)
10. Enhancement of gaseous and nutrient exchange at the tissue level (Barney et al., 1969; Editorial: Exercise, 1977)

People who engage in vigorous exercise tend to look better. They have an improved complexion, better posture, and their physiques begin to approach the Greco-Roman standard. Many individuals who exercise regularly report afterwards that they have feelings of euphoria, relaxation, and tranquility.

Exercises geared to prevent cardiac disease must enhance cardiovascular fitness. A few of the better-known programs that follow that principle are (1) the Royal Canadian Air Force Exercise Program, (2) the West Point fitness conditioning program, and (3) Kenneth Cooper's program, *Aerobics*. The premise behind all of these programs is that the heart and lungs must be effectively stimulated. According to the West Point program, the exercise should elevate the heart rate to about 70 percent of the maximum rate for the particular age, e.g. 134 to 142 for ages eighteen to twenty-nine and 99 to 105 for ages seventy to seventy-nine. The length of the exercise period depends upon the individual's condition. Generally, if the heart rate is maintained between 60 and 70 percent of maximum for the age-group, the exercise can be continued at that pace until the individual feels winded (usually between five and twelve minutes).

According to Cooper, the exercise should raise the heart rate up to an average minimum of 150 beats per minute (varies with age and condition), and the beneficial results begin about five minutes after the exercise starts. If the particular exercise is not vigorous enough to maintain an average heart rate of 150 beats per minute, but it still is demanding of oxygen, then the exercise should be continued for a considerably longer period than five minutes. The actual time depends upon the amount of oxygen consumed.

It is essential that a gradual warm-up period precede any strenuous exercise. Similarly, there should be a gradual tapering-off period. Good, vigorous exercises are running, jogging, swimming, jumping rope, and stationary bike riding. Participant sports and activities that contain sustained periods of vigorous exercise are handball, basketball, squash, racquetball, and dancing (Box 6-19). It is important that all dentists have a thorough medical examination, including a cardiovascular stress test, before beginning any strenuous exercise routine (Box 6-20 and Fig. 6-3).

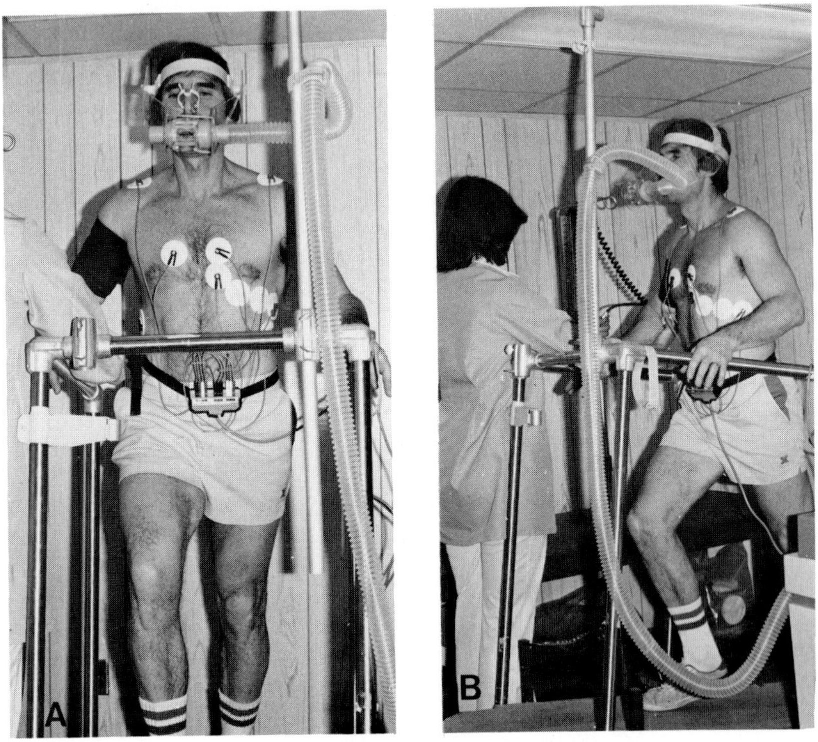

Figure 6-3. The senior author is shown undergoing the cardiovascular stress test. (*A*) The treadmill is horizontal. (*B*) The treadmill is inclined.

Box 6-19: The Aerobic Scale

Cooper (1968, 1977) has numerically rated different activities for their Aerobic value. He suggests working up to 30 points per week with this system. Some 30-point activities are (1) running 1.5 miles within twelve minutes, four times per week; (2) swimming 700 yards within fifteen minutes, five times per week; (3) cycling 6 miles within nineteen minutes, five times per week; (4) running in place for twenty minutes at 70 to 80 steps per minute, four times per week; (5) walking for 3 miles within forty-one minutes, five times per week; (6) playing squash or handball for fifty minutes (not including rest breaks), four times per week.

Box 6-20: The Stress Test

The condition of the heart, blood vessels, and the respiratory system is determined by the cardiovascular stress test. Subjects for the stress test are provided by referral from physicians after a preliminary medical examination (usually includes blood tests, blood pressure, and chest x-ray). At the testing center, a cardiologist reexamines the patient before beginning the stress test. (Tests taken include the resting electrocardiogram [EKG]; heart rate; and blood pressure.)

The stress test is usually taken by three groups of subjects: (1) patients suspected of having cardiovascular abnormalities, (2) individuals over thirty-five years of age who want a determination of their cardiovascular condition, and (3) people who are eager to have their physical fitness tested.

There are four measures of fitness examined: (1) EKG, (2) heart rate, (3) blood pressure, and (4) energy expenditure (O_2 consumption and CO_2 eliminated). The subject is "hooked up" and walks on a treadmill (it usually runs between 2 to 3 miles per hour) while his responses are fed into recording and viewing devices (Fig. 6-3*A*). The cardiologist observes the patient as well as the machines. As the test continues, the treadmill is gradually inclined (in order to increase the resistance and thus challenge the patient (Fig. 6-3*B*).

The stress test is continued until the subject achieves a target heart rate of 75 to 90 percent of his predicted maximum (based on a chart with values keyed to age and sex, e.g. maximum at age forty-five for males is 175. Depending on the patient's condition and the cardiologist's determination, the test is continued or terminated.

Some factors that help in determining at which point to end the test are (1) a fall in the O_2 retention of the lungs to 3 percent or less (about 5% is considered normal); (2) the heart rate exceeds 90 percent; (3) the blood pressure rises to too high a level (a gradual increase is considered normal); (4) serious EKG abnormalities are detected; (5) the patient's legs become fatigued; and (6) the patient reports that he can no longer continue (usually due to shortness of breath).

The patient is monitored as the test is gradually terminated. It is expected that within five minutes, blood pressure and pulse rate should return to resting levels. The results of the stress test are used to determine (1) the possible presence of cardiovascular disease (it is generally a good diagnostic test, but some diseased people may "pass" the test, and some healthy individuals may show occasional abnormalities); and (2) the level of cardiovascular fitness, which is a basis for tailoring an individual exercise training program.

The test is generally given in two sessions. The first hour is used as a diagnostic and get-acquainted session. The combination of the treadmill, the respiratory mask, the blood pressure cuff, and the EKG leads can induce anxiety and raise resting values. Hence, the preliminary visit helps overcome apprehension and acts to control for psychological artifacts. Including the preparatory and concluding phases, the sessions take approximately two hours. The usual cost is about $200, and comprehensive medical plans generally cover most of the fee. (Courtesy of Ms. Joan Carter and the staff of the Anthropometrics Heart Clinic, 56 Haddon Avenue, Haddonfield, New Jersey.)

Aside from the cardiovascular need for vigorous exercise, moderate activity performs other functions useful for the average dentist:

1. Combined with sensible eating and drinking, exercise tones the muscles and aids in maintenance of proper weight.
2. Proper exercise can help prevent back problems, and there are exercises useful to treat minor back conditions. For instance, pressing weights behind the back can maintain good posture and counteract the tendency of dentists to bend while working (Fig. 6-4). An exercise that can be useful in treating minor back problems is shown in Figure 6-5 (Barney et al., 1969; Kaplan, 1973; Lear, 1977; Norris, 1977).
3. Although golf and doubles tennis are not considered to be particularly effective for cardiovascular fitness, the activities are beneficial for good companionship. Talking to friends can help reduce psychological burdens.
4. Exercise can prevent cramps and pooling of blood that

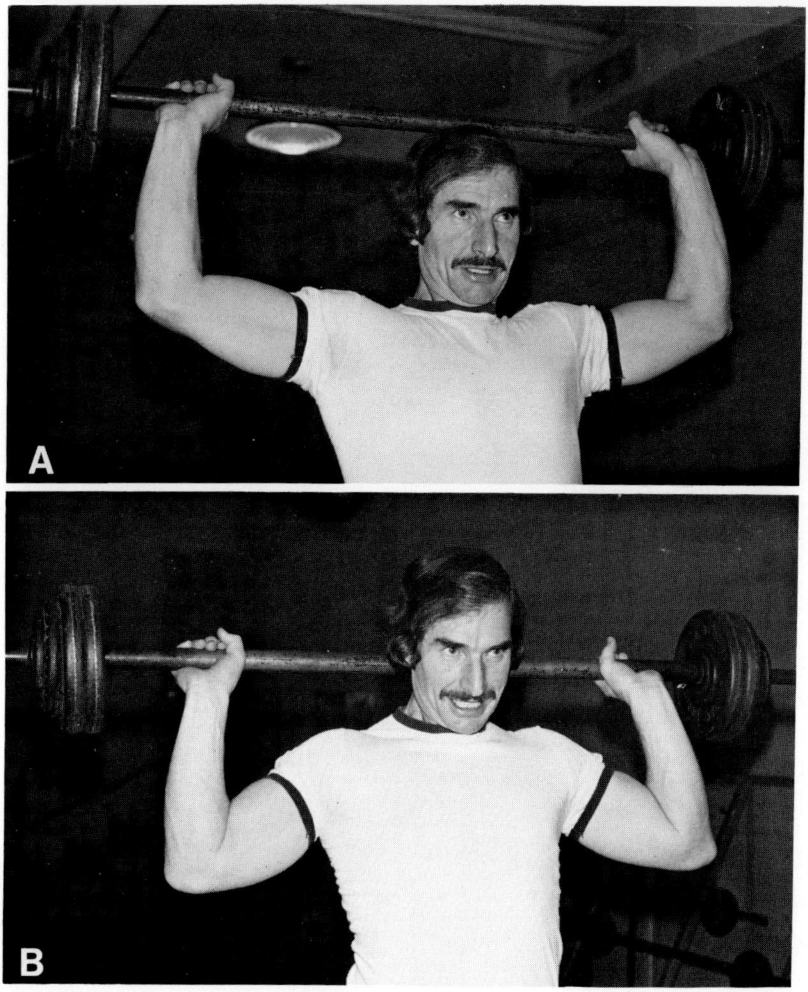

Figure 6-4. The senior author (a former intercollegiate weightlifting champion) demonstrates the press behind the neck. (*A*) The weight had been pressed to its maximum height and is now seen as it is being lowered behind the neck. The legs are planted firmly on the ground, about 15 inches apart. The buttocks are tensed. (*B*) The weight is now seen as it approaches its lowest point, slightly above the rear of the neck. Ten to fifteen repetitions of this exercise are recommended, provided that the individual has medical clearance.

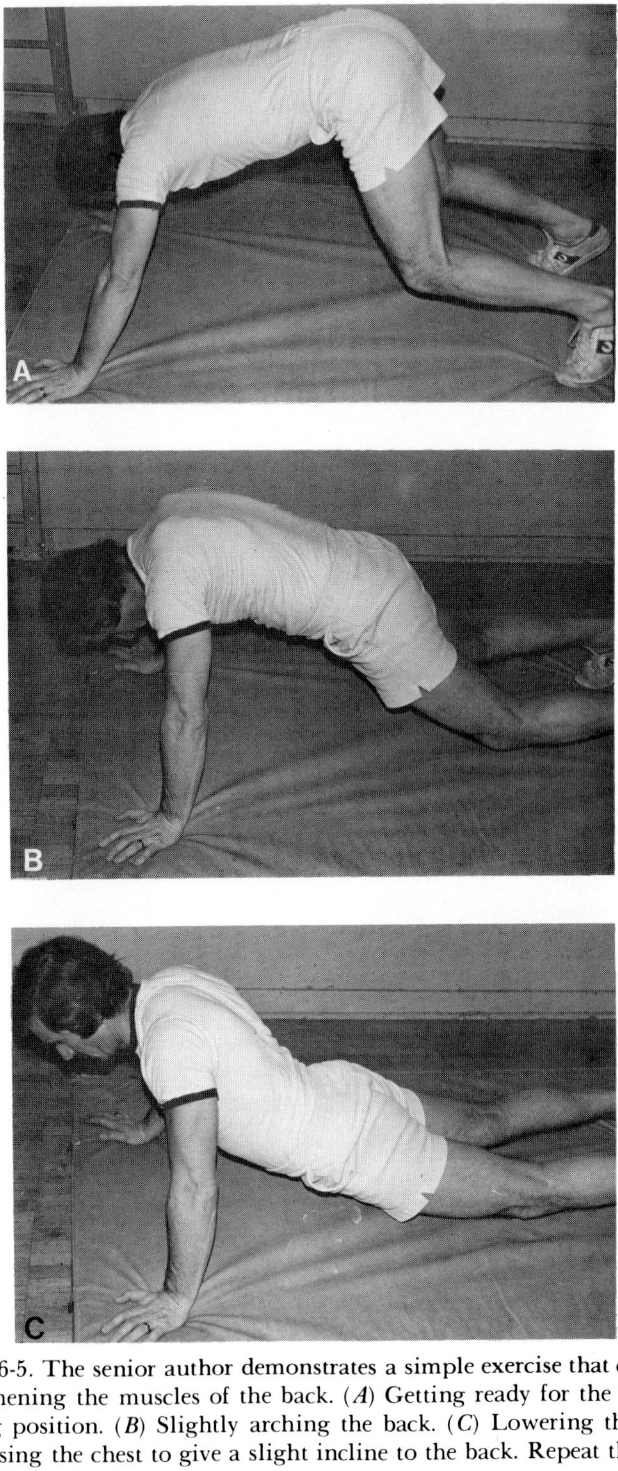

Figure 6-5. The senior author demonstrates a simple exercise that can help in strengthening the muscles of the back. (*A*) Getting ready for the "all-fours" starting position. (*B*) Slightly arching the back. (*C*) Lowering the buttocks and raising the chest to give a slight incline to the back. Repeat this exercise six times.

may occur from lack of movement and sitting or standing for long periods of times, i.e. for the prevention of varicosities. Hence, dentists should do simple exercises during working hours (Fig. 6-6).

5. The improvement in muscle and bone strength from lifting weights (or other strength-building exercises) can allow for greater ability to cope with physical stressors, i.e. they help in the "fight" stress response.

6. Fast reflex activities, such as Ping-Pong®, may aid one in escaping from physical stressors, i.e. they help in the "flight" stress response.

7. Strong muscles and bones decrease the body's vulnera-

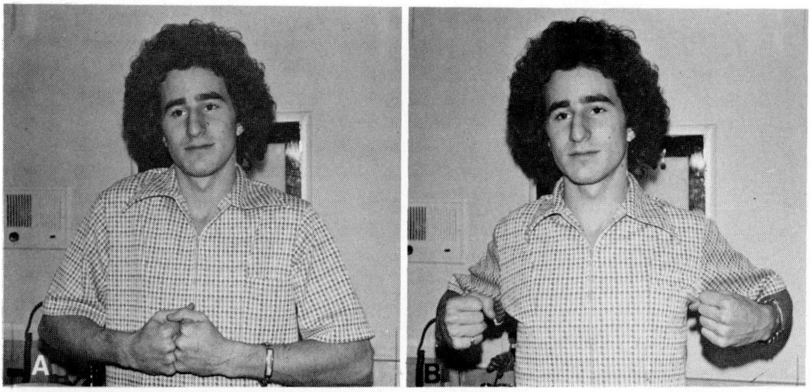

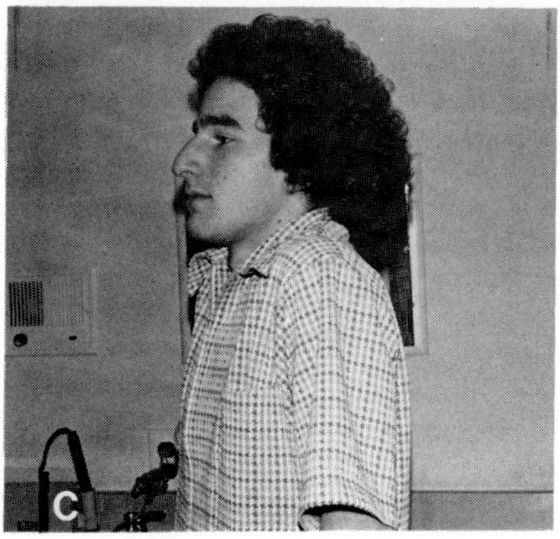

Figure 6-6 *A-C*. Simple exercises that can be done during the working day to improve circulation and prevent cramps. (Adapted from C. Norris: Is your back biting back? *Dent Manag, 17(9)*:57, 1977.) (*A*) Arms bent at the elbow and fists pushed against each other. (*B*) Arms separated and elbows forced backward as back is arched. Repeat several times. (*C*) The shoulders are shrugged forward and then backward. This exercise is good for the upper back and neck. Repeat several times.

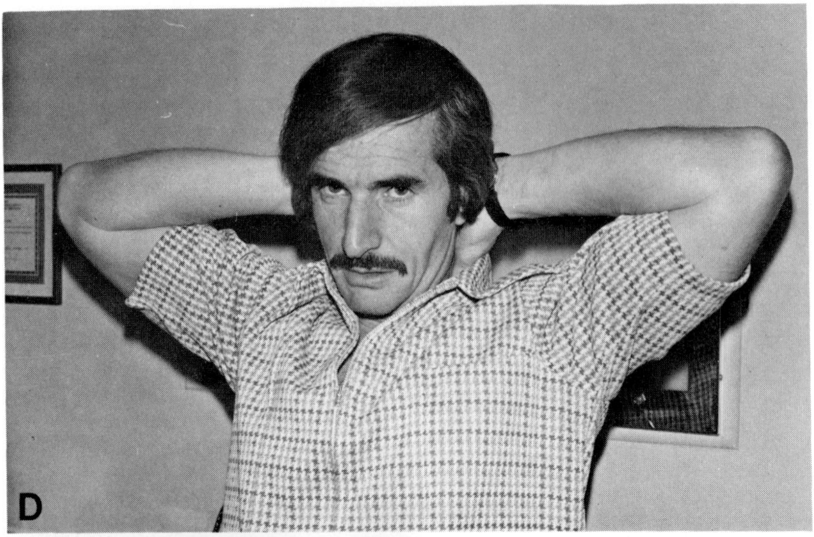

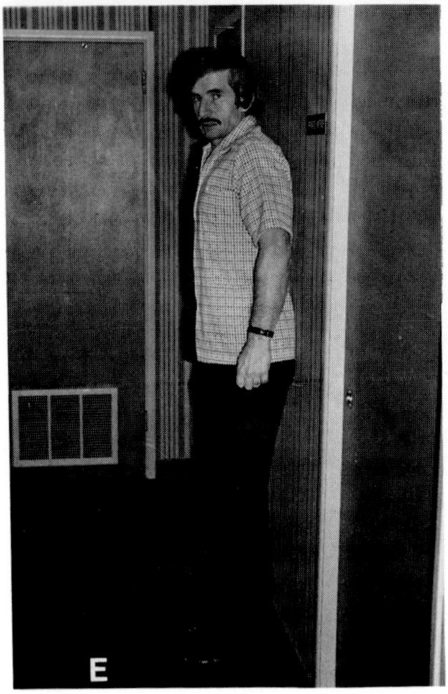

Figure 6-6 *D-E.* (*D*) A chest muscle-stimulating exercise. The hands are grasped behind the neck; the elbows are pulled backward and then brought forward. Repeat several times. (*E*) Toe raises. To increase calf muscle circulation, rise all the way up and then come completely down. Ten to fifteen repetitions are adequate. (*A-C*) Demonstrated by B. Morse. (*D, E*) Demonstrated by D. R. Morse.

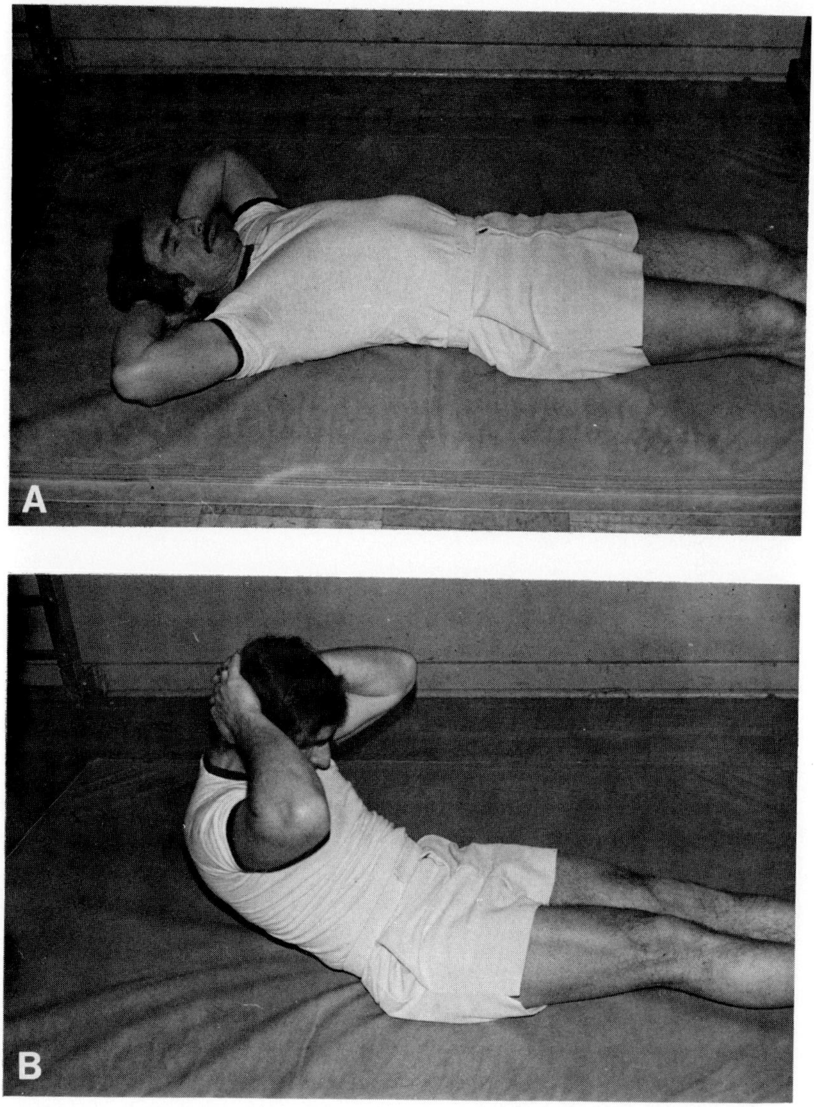

Figure 6-7 *A-B*. Abdominal muscle-strengthening exercises. (*A, B*) For the upper abdominals. (*A*) Lying on mat with hands clasped behind neck. (*B*) Sitting up halfway while keeping the legs straight on the ground.

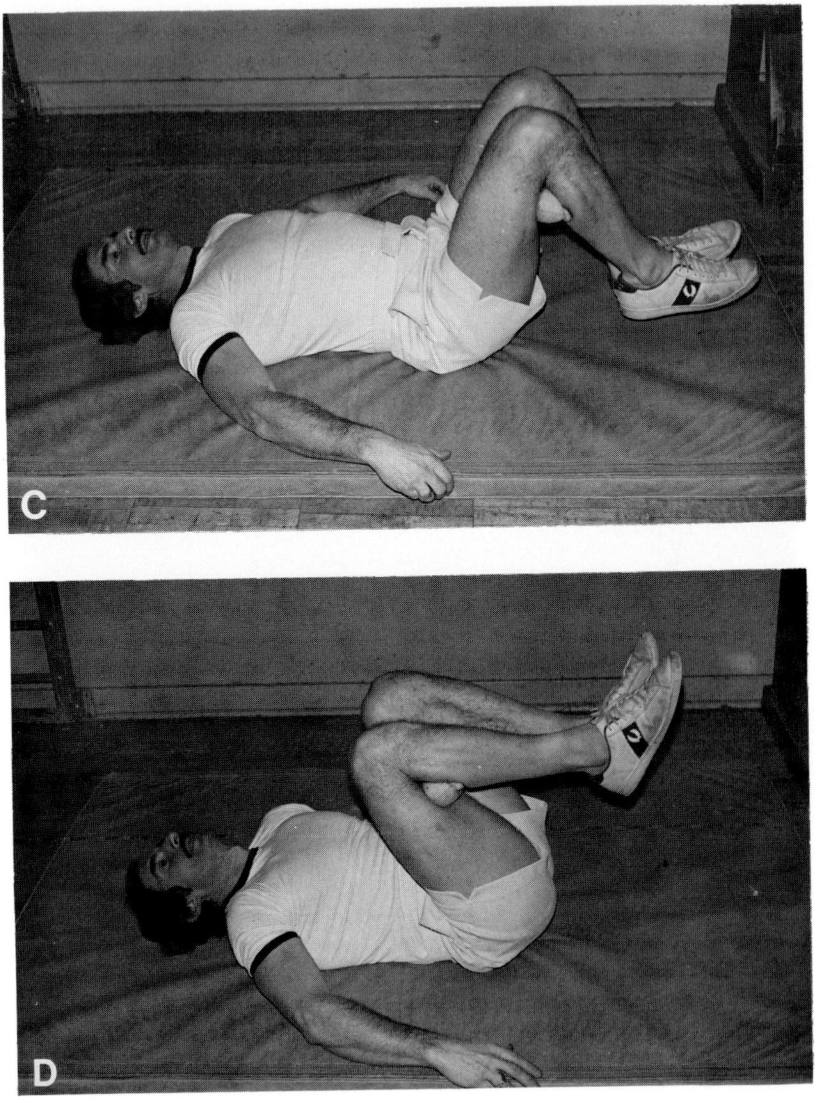

Figure 6-7 *C-D*. For the lower abdominals. (*C*) A sneaker is placed between bent knees, to help keep legs together (*D*) The bent legs are raised simultaneously while the upper body remains flat on the mat. This should be repeated ten to fifteen times.

bility to injury.

8. Strong abdominal muscles give better support for internal organs (typical abdominal exercises are shown in Figure 6-7).

9. Exercise not only increases strength and reflexes, it also increases energy and reduces fatigue. This allows a dentist to do his daily physical and mental work and still feel refreshed at the end of the day.

10. Regular exercise is beneficial for people who have trouble sleeping; simple stretching can help one arise easier in the morning (Fig. 6-8).

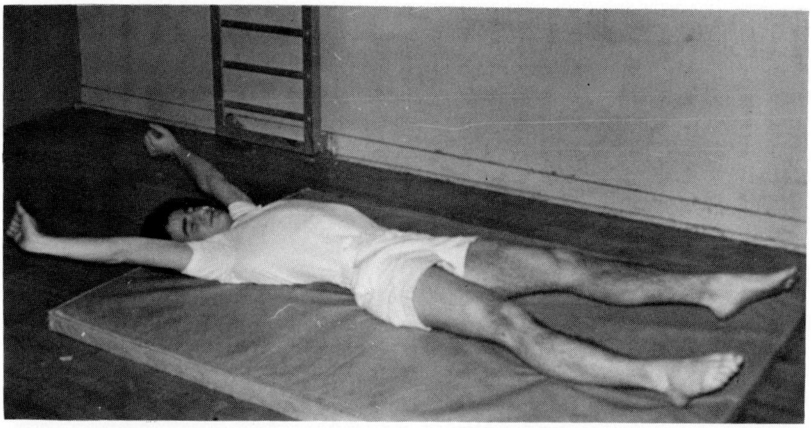

Figure 6-8. The full-body awakening stretch is demonstrated by B. Morse.

11. With respect to the increased circulation to all parts of the body, exercise can improve mental functioning simply as a result of the improved cerebral circulation.

12. Finally, exercise can induce or be combined with meditation (Box 6-21).

Box 6-21: Running Meditation

Earl Solomon (1977) has devised the *running meditation response*. It is a combination of slow, long-distance running with TM. He makes the following observations: (1) The runner experiences addiction, usually in two to four months. (2) The runner benefits physically as well as emotionally. (3)

The runner is totally vigilant and attentive, and his eyes remain open most of the time. (4) If carried out an hour at a time, there is vigorous and rhythmic contraction as well as relaxation of the large muscles of the trunk and legs. (5) The runner practices a special breathing technique.

Keeping the eyes open requires energy expenditure. Dyreke Spino (Bricklin, 1978) advocates semi-eye closure during running to induce greater relaxation. In using this method, the eyelids are relaxed until the eyes are almost closed. It is still possible to see through the slits, but the view is seen to be one of softness and restfulness.

Bill Gordon ran with his eyes completely closed. He reported that in the beginning it was "eerie" and frightening, but it soon became exhilarating. He felt a heightened awareness of his entire body (Bricklin, 1978).

With reduced vision in the first method and eyes closed in the modifications, it should be obvious that there be no obstacles or distractions in the running path. It is reported that one runner who did not exercise the caution called for in such a situation ran into a tree.

A clinical study has shown that exercise is beneficial for practicing dentists (Box 6-22).

Box 6-22: The Physically Fit Dentist

John Howard and his associates found that "for dentists, exercise not only helps work off the tensions of the job but gives a secondary payoff by improving one's physical condition and thereby his ability to cope with job pressures as they occur. . . Those participants who attempt to exercise suffer fewer than half the stress symptoms reported by the nonexercisers. . . Those who made an attempt to get at least a minimum amount of exercise showed a significantly higher physical work capacity" (Howard et al., 1976).

Laughing and Crying

Laughing and crying may be considered responses to stressors. Undoubtedly, there is a beneficial release in expressing these emotions. It is better not to inhibit the crying or laughing responses than to allow a buildup of psychological stressors, such as frustration and guilt. In view of the overwhelming number of stressors in the dental situation, the dentist should permit himself and his staff to smile, laugh, or cry as the circumstances warrant.

Pacing and Rocking

Some people pace up and down, apparently for no purpose, when they are under stress. In similar situations, others may rock, sew, or knit, e.g. the ex-football star Rosey Grier does needlepoint. These actions help calm apprehension and act as an outlet for the stress response.

Talking and Whistling

Some people talk to themselves when they are in trouble; some talk to others and try to "talk themselves out of trouble"; others scream or shout; still others whistle to relieve their anxieties. But sometimes there are no answers forthcoming; if this is the case, it may be time to seek aid.

Consultation

If the standard methods are tried and an individual still finds that he cannot cope, then he might turn to someone else for help. The dentist should first try his spouse, friends, and clergyman, and if none of these confidants can help, then he should seek professional assistance.

Admitting that one needs help is not a sign of weakness, any more than going to a dentist to take care of a toothache is an admission of "weak" teeth. Psychologists and psychiatrists are trained to help, so their counsel should be sought.* Psychotherapeutic methods that can be used to cope with anxiety and

---

*Confidential referrals may be made by the family physician or local professional societies and schools.

depression include psychoanalysis, client-centered psychotherapy, and behavioral therapies, e.g. assertiveness training and behavioral modification.

Group therapy may be a more effective method for some people to cope with stressors, and it should be considered. It may be that an individual is more comfortable in sharing his problems with others who have similar problems. There are various approaches that range from simple group psychotherapy to eclectic encounter groups. The many groups and courses combine in one form or another such techniques as relaxation, exercise, assertiveness training, transactional analysis, sensory deprivation, "brainwashing," and "touching and feeling." Some of the popular psychotherapies are Gestalt, EST (Erhard Seminar Training), Esalen, Reality, Psycho-cybernetics, Rational-Emotive, Silva Mind Control, psychodrama, and primal scream therapy. Another approach that may be taken is family therapy, in which the practitioner shares his problems in sessions with his family and the therapist. Some of the methods are quite demanding or even scientifically unsound, and an individual should check them out before he becomes involved.*

Summary

It can be seen that there are a number of approaches that a dentist can take to cope with the stressors of dentistry. It is believed that a sound mind in a sound body is the key to successful coping with life. Smoking, drinking, overeating, and drug intake may be temporarily effective but are self-defeating in the long run. A period should be set aside each day for relaxation, mental-preparation, exercise, and diversion. Most important, the dentist should make every attempt to enjoy not only the few hours of leisure set aside but also the many hours of work.

---

*Information may be obtained from local psychological and clinical hypnosis associations.

TREATING STRESS-RELATED CONDITIONS

Introduction

The stress-related conditions range from malaise through coronary artery disease to suicide. For each symptom and disease, there are specific treatments. There are also nonspecific therapies for the underlying stress. These therapies cover (1) behavior modification; (2) relaxation therapy; (3) rest; (4) antianxiety agents; and (5) exercise.

Symptoms and Diseases

In this section, the treatment of stress-related symptoms is considered first. Stress-related diseases are then covered, beginning with the most significant: coronary artery disease.

Symptoms

For each of the stress-related symptoms discussed in Chapter 4, there are specific medical treatments. The nonspecific remedies pertaining to these symptoms are discussed:

1. MALAISE: Malaise is a vague feeling of bodily discomfort that can occur with or without disease. Use of the relaxation response is often effective in changing malaise to euphoria.

2. PAIN: If pain is related to psychological stressors that result in muscle tension, then meditation, self-hypnosis, and biofeedback are generally effective. Moderate exercise is also helpful in decreasing tension-related pain.

3. FATIGUE: In Chapter 1, several terms used in physics and biology were discussed, e.g. stress, pressure, and tension. Another term of interest is fatigue. In its physics use, *fatigue* is a weakness in a metal, wood, or other material that results from prolonged stress. Biologically, there are four definitions of fatigue: (a) Physical fatigue is exhaustion resulting from muscular overexertion. (b) Fatigue of individual muscle units results from the accumulation of lactic acid. (c) Mental fatigue

is severe mental weariness resulting from either excessive mental or physical exertion. (d) In Hans Selye's general adaptation syndrome, fatigue (or exhaustion) is the third and final stage in which the body can no longer adjust physiologically and is likely to succumb to serious disease.

The exhaustion stage is a more serious state than any of the other three kinds of fatigue, and it generally results from unrelenting stressors. To combat such fatigue, it is essential to get away from the stress situation. For instance, if the stressor is infection, the person might have to be treated with massive antibiotic therapy and given intravenous fluids and bed rest.

Muscle fatigue can be treated by complete rest of the particular muscle group to allow for removal of the accumulated lactic acid and reformation of muscle glycogen (needed for energy). The fatigue from exercise is generally a pleasant feeling, unless one is out-of-condition and feels like collapsing. For the conditioned athlete, a few hours of rest rejuvenates the fatigued body. For the out-of-shape individual, several days of rest may be necessary for recuperation.

For mental fatigue, the best therapy is simply to stop the current mental activity and relax either by watching TV, listening to soft music, or practicing the relaxation response. If mental fatigue results from working too hard or too long at one activity, such as at the dental chair, then for the protection of both the patient and dentist, it is essential to stop the activity. If the fatigue continually recurs, the dentist should consider (a) shorter working hours, (b) alternating treatment procedures and sequences, (c) taking a two-hour lunch, (d) taking regular relaxation breaks during working hours, and (e) going on a vacation.

4. WEAKNESS: Weakness occurs from overexertion, being out-of-condition, or being exposed to severe stressors such as infective microbes. Having adequate sleep, a good diet, regular exercise, and frequent relaxation breaks can help prevent this stress outcome. Rest, relaxation, an adequate fluid intake, and moderate exercise may be of help in the treatment of weakness.

5. CHILLS: Chills can occur from being underclothed or from infectious disease. Wearing warm clothing and avoiding drafts are good preventive measures. With good resistance, one becomes better able to cope with microbial stressors that can cause chills. Treatment includes fluids, rest, and warm clothing.

6. SWEATING: Sweating may result from strenuous exercise, from taking a steam bath, or as a sequel to infectious microbes. The sweating from exercise or baths can be taken care of by a shower and towel drying. Sweating from disease is partly controlled by loosening clothing, drying with towels, and cool drinks.

7. HIGH FEVER: Body temperature tends to rise with exercise, steam baths, and disease. The treatment aims at cooling down the body with such things as cold baths and an alcohol rub.

8. INSOMNIA: Insomnia can result from physical and mental overexertion, psychological stressors, and disease. Treatment takes the form of "counting sheep," meditating while lying down, and drinking warm milk. Getting regular exercise helps prevent insomnia.

9. STOMACHACHE: Stomachache can result from eating foods that "don't agree," traumatic injury, and disease. Avoidance of known indigestible foods is a good preventive measure. Bed rest and relaxation are usually helpful for treatment.

10. APPETITE LOSS: Appetite loss may be a manifestation of poor body condition or disease. With regular exercise and planned periods of relaxation, appetite generally improves. With respect to microbial disease, after the infection is successfully treated, the appetite soon returns to normal.

11. DIZZINESS: Dizziness can result from head injuries, psychological stressors, and disease. When one is dizzy, one should move about cautiously, avoid any sudden movements, and lie down at the earliest opportunity. A few deep breaths may help.

12. FAINTING: Fainting occurs from cerebral anoxia. It can result from psychological stressors or disease. Oxygen is the treatment of choice. Blood flow to the head region is vital, and the individual's body should not be raised to a sitting position.

Coronary Artery Disease

As far as specific treatment is concerned, the particular condition and the attending physician determine the appropriate measures to be taken. For prevention, it seems to make sense to (1) cut down on high-cholesterol foods, e.g. milk, butter, eggs, and beef; (2) reduce high-carbohydrate consumption; (3) decrease salt intake; (4) quit smoking; (5) exercise frequently; (6) have regular periods of deep relaxation; (7) try to avoid or evade stressors; and (8) learn to better cope with stressors. From the stress aspect, all of the factors mentioned above are even more important to follow after one has suffered a heart attack. However, the exercise regimen has to be carefully monitored.

For treatment of hypertension, there are specific antihypertensive drugs that are quite effective. One group of drugs that is currently popular is the *β-blockers*. Beta-blockers, such as propranolol, act to inhibit many of the actions of the sympathetic nervous system. They specifically block the endings of the norepinephrine nerve fibers. The β-blockers also inhibit palpitations. Propranolol is used to treat hypertension, cardiac arrhythmias, tachycardia, and anxiety.

Herbert Benson has pioneered in the use of meditation as a method to decrease blood pressure for hypertensives. Several studies have shown that meditation, hypnosis, relaxation therapy, and biofeedback can lower blood pressure, decrease cardiac arrhythmias, reduce heart rate, and relieve anxiety (Benson, 1977; Morse, 1977). Even when meditation is effective, it is still usually necessary for the patients to continue their medications.

Miscellaneous Diseases

For the many other stress-related diseases, a discussion of the specific treatments is beyond the scope of this book. Nevertheless, as Hans Selye (1976) has shown, stress is the underlying factor in almost every disease. Hence, all of the methods of prevention and coping with stress discussed in this chapter are appropriate to prevent the onset of a given disease and to decrease the severity and aftereffects, particularly if the disease is already present. Psychotherapy is one method that is not often considered in the treatment of stress-related diseases. Yet, it may be very effective (Box 6-23).

Box 6-23: Psychotherapy For The Gut

A study of two groups of patients with colitis was reported by Adelle Davis (1965). Group A patients were given a carefully controlled diet along with the usual required medications. Group B patients, who were judged to have more severe cases of colitis, received no specific diets and were not put on medications. However, they received three months of frequent, sympathetic psychotherapy. Greater improvement, less hemorrhaging, less requirement for surgical intervention, and fewer deaths were found with the group B patients.

Another interesting finding regarding mental attitude and disease is worth reporting. As discussed in Chapter 4, many cancer patients had feelings of anxiety, depression, and hopelessness prior to the onset of their disease. There is some circumstantial evidence that being happy and positive in one's mental outlook may help prevent or ameliorate cancer. It has been observed that individuals who have had spontaneous remissions of cancer generally can be classified as having had a strong will to live; they have been reported to have had a more positive outlook on life (not being depressed), as compared to those who succumbed to cancer (Arehart-Treichel, 1977; Box 6-24).

Box 6-24: Mental Conquest of Cancer

Although it was not a controlled study, Carl Simonton has reported on several cases in which a mental technique was used along with conventional therapy to induce apparent complete remission of cancer. The mental technique consisted of relaxation, meditation, and visualization. The patients were asked to visualize their cancer, i.e. as a cauliflower or a water-filled balloon. Then, if they were having radiation therapy, they were told to picture the rays striking and shrinking the cancerous growth. If they were receiving oral drugs, they were asked to visualize the pills dissolving and then poisoning the cancer cells. They were also asked to picture their white blood cells attacking and destroying the malignant cells.

Simonton found that those patients who had successful remissions were able to visualize well and actively partook in their treatment. They looked on life in a positive way; their outlook was bright and cheerful. Those who succumbed were uncooperative, e.g. would not stop smoking, and had a bleak mental outlook (Halsell, 1976).

Disorders

In Chapter 4, the various disorders that can befall the dental practitioner, ranging from drinking to divorce, were evaluated. Quite often depression leads to other problems, such as drinking, drug addiction, divorce, practice failure, and suicide. Hence, depression should be prevented or treated. The various methods of coping discussed in this chapter should help in this regard. However, it is most important that the depression-prone dentist seeks counsel. Beginning in dental school and continuing throughout his career, psychological counseling should be made available to each dentist. Dentists have to learn to share their problems. When this is appreciated, it will facilitate solving the problem of stress-related disorders.

Summary

Dentistry is a major health profession that ranks high in the public opinion. However, all too often the individual patient regards treatment as a necessary evil. The patient's apprehensions add to the stressful nature of the dentist's work. Hence, the end result is that dentistry is a potentially stressful occupation. There are many ways to deal with the stressors of dentistry; all are not effective for everyone. Those of major importance may be stated as follows: (1) Avoid those stressful situations that you can. (2) Be prepared for those that you cannot avoid. (3) Have regular daily periods of deep relaxation. (4) Practice moderation in eating, drinking, smoking, drug intake, and sleeping. (5) Exercise regularly. (6) Have a means of diversion. (7) Do not neglect the importance of consultations.

REFERENCES

Anderson, J. L. and Cohen, M.: *The West Point Fitness and Diet Book*. New York, Rawson Associates, 1977.

Arehart-Treichel, J.: Can your personality kill you? *New York Magazine, 10:*26, Nov. 28, 1977.

Barney, V. S., Hirst, C. C., and Jensen, C. R.: Conditioning Exercises: Exercises to Improve Body Form and Function, 2nd ed. St. Louis, Mosby, 1969.

Beane, M.: Longer life? It's your decision. *Prevention, 26(2):*42, 1974.

Belloc, N. B.: Relationship of health practices and mortality. *Prev Med, 2:*67, 1973.

Benson, H.: Systemic hypertension and the relaxation response. *N Engl J Med, 296:*1152, 1977.

Benson, H., Beary, J. F., and Carol, M. P.: The relaxation response. *Psychiatry, 37:*37, 1974.

Blake, D.: Is it too easy to finance that new practice? *Dent Manag, 17(11):*57, 1977.

Borland, L. C.: Letter to editor: Dentistry was the right choice. *Dent Surv, 53(4):*23, 1977.

Bosco, D.: Nutrition under the knife. Part II. *Prevention, 30(1):*83, 1978.

Boston Collaborative Drug Surveillance Program: Coffee drinking and acute myocardial infarction. *Lancet, 2:*1278, 1972.

Boszormenyi-Nagy, I. and Framo, J. L.: *Intensive Family Therapy*. New York, Hoeber Medical Division, Har-Row, 1965.

Bourquin, A. and Musmanno, E.: Preliminary report on the effect of smoking on the ascorbic acid content of whole blood. *Am J Dig Dis, 20:*75, 1953.

Bricklin, M.: Trade yourself in for a new model. *Prevention, 29(2):*32, 1977.

____ : This year make time for fun. *Prevention, 30(1):*32, 1978.

Carrington, P.: *Freedom in Meditation: Getting the Most Out of Meditating*. New York, Anch. Doubleday, 1977; Doubleday paperbacks, 1978.

Castleton, V. I.: Use essential oils to get more from a massage. *Prevention, 29(2):*143, 1977.

Chernov, M. S., Hale, H. W., Jr., and Wood, M.: Prevention of stress ulcers. *Am J Surg, 122:*674, 1971.

Cinotti, W. R., Grieder, A., and Springob, H. K.: *Applied Psychology in Dentistry,* 2nd ed. St. Louis, Mosby, 1972, pp. 253-259.

Collison, D. R.: Cardiological applications of the control of the autonomic nervous sytem by hypnosis. *Am J Clin Hypn, 12:*150, 1970.

Cooper, K. H.: *Aerobics.* New York, M. Evans and Co., Inc., 1968.

——: *The Aerobics Way.* New York, M. Evans and Co., 1977.

Corsini, R. J.: *Methods of Group Psychotherapy.* New York, Blakiston, 1957.

Daniels, L. K.: The treatment of psycho-physiological disorders and severe anxiety by behavior therapy, hypnosis and transcendental meditation. *Am J Clin Hypn, 17:*267, 1975.

Davis, A.: *Let's Get Well.* New York, Harcourt Brace and World, Inc., 1965.

Deabler, H. L., Fidel, B. S., Dillenkoffer, R. L., and Elder, S. T.: The use of relaxation and hypnosis in lowering high blood pressure. *Am J Clin Hypn, 16:*75, 1973.

Dennis, M. J.: Tuition is high at Georgetown, but financial aid meets 85 percent of students' need. *Dent Manag, 17(11):*54, 1977.

Dunlap, J. E.: *Serving in Dentistry: The Sources of Stress.* Tulsa, PPC Books, 1977.

Dyce, J. M.: *Stress and Decision-making in the Dental Practice.* Chicago, Quintessence Publ. Co., 1973.

Editorial: Beta-blockers in anxiety and stress. *Br Med J, 2:*415, 1976.

Editorial: Caffeine toxicity. *Exec Fitness Newsletter,* Sample Issue 3, 1977.

Editorial: Dentists, other health professionals lead smoking decline. *Dent Surv, 53(12):*63, 1977.

Editorial: The dentist's personal health problems — And some remedies. *Dent Surv, 52(2):*12, 1976.

Editorial: Exercise after 30. *Exec Fitness Newsletter,* Sample Issue 2, 1977.

Editorial: Loneliness really can kill you. *Philadelphia Evening Bulletin,* 23, Dec. 15, 1977.

Editorial: Medicine: Coronary curb: Bully for the strenuous life. *Time, 110(24):*80, Dec. 12, 1977.

Editorial: Pantothenate — The anti-stress vitamin. *Prevention, 29(11):*127, 1977.

Editorial: The penalty of sin. *Exec Fitness Newsletter,* Sample Issue 1, 1977.

Eliot, R. S.: Stress and cardiovascular disease. *Eur J Cardiol, 5(2):*97, 1977.

Feltman, J.: A nutritional shield against the arrows of stress. *Prevention, 28(9):*88, 1976.

——: Raise your serum fun level. *Prevention, 29(7):*148, 1977.

Foley, W. J.: Stress from many sources affects your health and well being. *Dent Stud, 55(8):*34, 1977.

French, A. P. and Tupin, J. P.: Therapeutic application of a simple relaxation method. *Am J Psychother, 28:*282, 1974.

Friedman, H. and Taub, H. A.: The use of hypnosis and biofeedback procedures for essential hypertension. *Int J Clin Exp Hypn, 25:*335, 1977.

Gallwey, W. T.: *The Inner Game of Tennis.* New York, Random, 1974.

Glass, D. C.: Stress, behavior patterns and coronary disease. *Am Sci, 65:*177, 1977.

Goleman, D.: Meditation helps break the stress spiral. *Psychol Today, 9(2):*82, 1976.

Gottlieb, B.: Release your tension with massage. *Prevention, 29(2):*134, 1977.

Green, D.: The class of '76: How well are they winging it? *Dent Manag, 17(12):*22, 1977.

Grzesiak, R. C.: Relaxation techniques in treatment of chronic pain. *Arch Phys Med Rehabil, 58:*270, 1977.

Halsell, G.: Mind over cancer. *Prevention, 28(1):*118, 1976.

Hilgard, E. R., Atkinson, R. C., and Atkinson, R. L.: Techniques of psychotherapy. In Hilgard, E. R. (Ed.): *Introduction to Psychology,* 6th ed. New York, HarBrace J, 1975, pp. 497-521.

Hodges, R. E.: The effect of stress on ascorbic acid metabolism in man. *Nutr Today, 5(1):*11, 1970.

Howard, J. H., Cunningham, D. A., Rechnitzer, P. A., and Goode, R. C.: Stress in the job and career of a dentist. *JADA, 93:*630, 1976.

Jackson, E. and Mealica, W. I., Jr.: Stress management and personal satisfaction in dental practice. *Dent Clin North Am, 21:*559, 1977.

Johnsen, J. and Johnsen, E.: For married students, it can't work without a lot of sharing. *Dent Manag, 17(11):*47, 1977.

Kaplan, D.: More on coping with posture-related backache. *Dent Surv, 49(5):*47, 1973.

Keys, A.: Coronary heart disease in seven countries. *Circulation (Suppl. 1), 41:*211, 1970.

Kinderlehrer, J.: Improve your moods with better diet. *Prevention, 25(2):*79, 1973.

Klumpp, T. G.: How much exercise to avoid heart attacks? *Med Times, 104(4):*64, 1976.

Kroger, W. S.: Nudism, Esalen, other therapy. *Osteopath Physician, 43(4):*98, Apr., 1976.

Lazarus, R. S.: *Coping With Stress: Effects on Somatic Illness, Morale, and Social Function.* Read before the Symposium on Stress and Behavioral Medicine. New York, Dec. 3-4, 1977.

Lear, L.: Here's help for your aching back. *Prevention, 29(2):*103, 1977.

Leff, D. N.: Stress-triggered organic disease in this year of economic anxiety. *Med World News, 16:*74, March 24, 1975.

Manber, M.: The medical effects of coffee. *Med World News, 17:*63, Jan. 26, 1976.

Mann, G. V.: Medical intelligence: Current concepts: Diet-heart: End of an era. *N Engl J Med, 297:*644, 1977.

Maugh, T. H., II.: Coffee and heart disease: Is there a link? *Science, 181:*534, 1973.

Morse, D. R.: *Clinical Endodontology: A Comprehensive Guide to Diagnosis,*

Treatment and Prevention. Springfield, Ill., Thomas, 1974, pp. 35-42, 395.

____ : Overcoming "practice stress" via meditation and hypnosis. *Dent Surv, 53(7)*:32, 1977.

____ : Variety, exercise, meditation can relieve practice stress. *Dent Stud, 56(3)*:26, 1977.

____ : General practice, specialty or teaching: Which one's for you? *Dent Manag, 18(6)*:In press, 1978.

National Clearing House for Smoking and Health and the National Cancer Institute: *Survey of Health Professionals: Smoking and Health, 1975,* U.S. Govt Print Office, Washington, D.C.

Norris, C.: Is your back biting back? *Dent Manag, 17(9)*:57, 1977.

Padus, E.: Easy yoga for everybody. *Prevention, 29(5)*:55, 1977.

Palmore, E. B.: Physical, mental, and social factors in predicting longevity. *Gerontologist, 9*:103, 1969.

Patel, C. and North, W. R. S.: Randomized controlled trial of yoga and biofeedback in management of hypertension. *Lancet, 2*:93, 1975.

Pollack, A. A., Case, D. B., Weber, M. A., and Laragh, J. H.: Limitations of transcendental meditation in the treatment of essential hypertension. *Lancet, 1*:71, 1977.

Reynolds, G. S.: The effects of stress upon problem solving. *J Gen Psychol, 62*:83, 1960.

Revelle, W., Amaral, P., and Turiff, S.: Introversion/extroversion, time stress and caffeine: Effect on verbal performance. *Science, 192*:149, 1976.

Rodale, R.: Mind power can relax you. *Prevention, 29(8)*:25, 1977.

Saikkonen, J.: Saunas. *Arch Phys Med Rehabil, 58(6)*:277, 1977.

Seifter, E.: Of stress, vitamin A, and tumors. *Science, 193*:74, 1976.

Selye, H.: Further thoughts on "stress without distress." *Med Times, 104(11)*:124, 1976.

Shaw, R. E.: Mercury is a hazard of your workplace. *Dent Stud, 55(8)*:26, 1977.

Sherlock, B. J. and Morris, R. T.: *Becoming a Dentist.* Springfield, Ill., Thomas, 1972.

Siegal, S.: *Dr. Siegal's Natural Fiber Permanent Weight-Loss Diet.* New York, Dial, 1975.

Solomon, E.: *Running and Meditation.* Read before the symposium on Meditation Related Therapies. St. Louis, Oct. 28-29, 1977.

Spilman, C.: Exercises for people who don't have the time. *Prevention, Pt. 1, 26(1)*:76; *Pt. 2, 26(2)*:127, 1974.

Stone, R. A. and DeLeo, J.: Psychotherapeutic control of hypertension. *N Engl J Med, 294*:80, 1976.

Sword, R. O.: Stress and suicide among dentists: Competitiveness and "being all things." *Dent Surv, 53(4)*:10, 1977.

Szorady, I.: Pantothenic acid: Experimental results and clinical observations. *Acta Paediatr Acad Sci Hung, 4*:73, 1963.

Taylor, C. B., Farquhar, J. W., Nelson, E., and Agras, S.: Relaxation therapy and high blood pressure. *Arch Gen Psychiatry, 34:*339, 1977.

Voss, L. and Shimoda, T.: Protect against free NO_2 in the operatory — For health's sake. *Dent Stud, 55(8):*62, 1977.

Walters, E.: How to live with failure and stress. *Dent Manag, 16(10):*20, 1976.

Weiss, C. M.: Variety is the spice of dentistry. *Dent Manag, 17(11):*15, 1977.

Weiss, T.: Biofeedback training for cardiovascular dysfunctions. *Med Clin North Am, 61:*913, 1977.

West, E.: Our search to know ourselves. *Sky, 5(5):*20, 1976.

Wheeler, A. C.: Try a tisane for tranquility: To the knowledgeable, herb teas are a source of serenity or stimulation, and always a flavor delight. *Prevention, 24(6):*142, 1972.

Whieldon, D.: Drinkers, addicts, depressives: What happens when they're doctors? *Pract Psychol Physicians, 4(11):*13, 1977.

Whiteside, D. F.: Here's what recent federal legislation may offer you in the way of financial aid. *Dent Manag, 17(11):*50, 1977.

Williams, R. J.: *Nutrition Against Disease: Environmental Prevention.* New York, Pitman, 1971.

Wolfe, R. C.: Little things I learned from four malpractice suits. *Dent Manag, 18(2):*21, 1978.

Worsham, J.: Secrets of looking and feeling younger. *Prevention, 25(2):*88, 1973.

Wyll, S. L.: Stress prevention in dentistry. *Dent Surv, 53(12):*57, 1977.

Yanovski, A. and Curtis, G. C.: Hypnosis and stress. *Am J Clin Hypn, 10:*149, 1968.

CHAPTER 7

PUTTING IT ALL TOGETHER

Conclusions are drawn and avenues of improvement are considered. Incorporation of stress-reducing and stress-coping methods into dental school and dental practice is examined.

INTRODUCTION

PRACTICE. Patience. Patients. Pride. Prestige. Profit. In Chapter 4, the six D's of stress-related disorders were presented. However, if dentists can learn to cope with the stress of dentistry, then the six P's might replace the six D's. For when one *p*ractices with skill, *p*atience, and empathy, the rewards can be appreciative *p*atients, *p*ride in one's work, *p*restige in the community, and a *p*rofitable *p*ractice.

CAPSULE COMMENT

The stress of dentistry is real, but it is probably part of the times. Citizens of the United States have witnessed catastrophic changes from the development of the atomic bomb to the invasion of outer space. We live with war and threats of war. Carcinogenic chemicals surround us, and a viable ecology is being threatened. Yet, we can travel halfway around the world in a day and enjoy the delights of a sauna bath in our homes.

It is up to all of us to change what we can, avoid what we cannot, and enjoy what we have. These principles certainly apply to dentistry. The public should be educated about the benefits of modern dentistry. Dentists should be free to practice at locations they choose and with patients who stand to benefit most from their services. To cope with the rigors of dentistry, dentists should be mentally prepared and physically fit. Adequate time should be set aside each day for rest, relaxation, proper nutrition, exercise, and diversion. Given these things, the practice of dentistry can be a challenge and a reward rather than a bore and a chore (Box 7-1).

Box 7-1: Forewarned and Forearmed

Miller and Dworkin (1977) found that "toughened-up" rats coped better; Szorady's (1963) nutritionally prepared mice were better reactors to stress; Benson (1977) showed that meditation decreased blood pressure; and studies by Belloc (1973) and Paffenberger (Editorial: Medicine: Coronary Curb, 1977) revealed that exercise is important in disease prevention.

These and other findings indicate people have a greater ability to manage stress if they (1) regularly practice the relaxation response, (2) have a positive mental outlook, (3) maintain a balanced diet, and (4) engage in a systematic exercise program.

An investigation by Vogel and his co-workers (1959) reinforces this concept. They found that subjects with high physiological reactivity performed in a superior manner, as compared to subjects with low physiological reactivity.

THE FUTURE

Besides providing opportunities to develop basic clinical skills, dental school and practice are geared to improve the techniques of dentistry. And, of course, without technical proficiency there would be no clinical advances. Yet, for the sake of the dentist's health, changes should occur.

Recognizing the limitations of time, money, and manpower, ideally such changes should occur before the student is admitted to dental school. Each prospective student should be evaluated psychologically as well as scholastically. This may involve psychological interviews in addition to filling out detailed questionnaires.

One possibility is the use of the stress interview. This interviewing technique was developed during World War II for selection and assignment of men by the Office of Strategic

Services (OSS). The stress interview helps in determining how well an individual can keep control of his resources while under severe psychological stressors. Such a procedure may help establish each student's stress level (safety zone) and perhaps help the admissions committee in the decision making processes.

In dental schools, provision should be made for stress management in the same way that provision is made for curriculum and clinical skills. Periods set aside each day for relaxation and exercise breaks can be envisioned. Facilities may include a small gymnasium, a sauna, and a room with comfortable chairs to allow for the practice of the relaxation response. These concepts may be considered visionary or idealistic, but industry already has seen the wisdom of such an approach for their employees.* It is ironic that the health professions should be lagging so far behind.

Students should have access to psychological consultations. Psychological consultation time should be built into the schedule so that students could be counseled before problems become unmanageable.

We should bring back into advanced education the joys children had in elementary school. Do you recall the times when you looked forward to gym and recess? Do you remember that the school counselor, as well as the school nurse, was readily available?

Regarding dental practice, changes should be contemplated with the dentists' physical and mental health kept in mind. When dental architects design an office, they should incorporate into the plan a small relaxation room and a small gym with an adjoining shower. From a narrow point of view, the cost might be considered prohibitive, but the long-term return in prevention and health is well worth the initial investment. Of course, simply having the facility is not sufficient: It must be used. The dentist should set aside time periods during each working day for exercise and relaxation. Practicing in this way should improve the dentist's mental outlook and physical

---

*For example, the Chase Manhattan Bank in New York employs comprehensive stress testing for its employees and also has a well-equipped gymnasium designated for employee use.

health, and might even make him more pleasant at the end of a hard day as he approaches home. In sum, it may be that a evaluation of priorities is called for by an enlightened dental community.

REFERENCES

Belloc, N. B.: Relationship of health practices and mortality. *Prev Med, 2:*63, 1973.

Benson, H.: Systemic hypertension and the relaxation response. *N Engl J Med, 296:*1152, 1977.

Editorial: Medicine: Coronary curb: Bully for the strenuous life. *Time, 110(24):*80, Dec. 12, 1977.

Miller, N. E. and Dworkin, B. R.: Effects of learning on visceral functions—Biofeedback. *N Engl J. Med, 296:*1274, 1977.

Office of Strategic Service Assessment: *Assessment of Men.* New York, HR&W, 1958.

Szorady, I.: Pantothenic acid: Experimental results and clinical observations. *Acta Paediatr Acad Sci Hung, 4:*73, 1963.

Vogel, W., Raymond, S., and Lazarus, R. S.; Intrinsic motivation and psychological stress. *J Abnorm Soc Psychol, 58:*225, 1959.

APPENDICES

Opening Our Mouths and Letting Our Teeth Show

APPENDIX 1

HOW WE DO IT

THE AUTHORS' PERSONAL METHODS OF COPING

One is a teacher and an endodontist; the other is a teacher and psychologist. They have written a dental text about stress and its management. The reader might rightfully wonder whether they practice what they preach. While they are not perfect models, they manage. In order to show this, their personal ways of coping are presented.

D. M.'s Story

LET us look at a typical Monday. After arising and taking care of necessities, the first stress-relieving method is undertaken. This is the morning meditation. Next is a short exercise period consisting of sit-ups, leg raises, and running in place for five minutes. Then, after washing and brushing, there is breakfast. An average breakfast starts with orange juice and a multiple vitamin-mineral supplement (including the potential antistress vitamins, B complex, C, and E). Next, I usually have a mixture of fortified skim milk (vitamins A and D added), cold cereal, e.g. Total®, bran, and wheat germ, and raisins. Then it is time for the drive to work. The stress level is raised by the heavy traffic and the generally depressing eight o'clock news. The stress level is somewhat decreased by listening to classical music (after the news).

The school day begins with an 8:30 to 10:00 immunology lecture. Coffee break is from 10:00 to 10:15. The usual bill of fare is hot tea and a granola bar. The remainder of the morning is taken up with the clinical evaluation of the first-year graduate students (the stress level decreases as the students get more proficient). Lunch is light; generally one of the fruit-flavored yogurts. Monday is a halfday at school; hence, about an hour after lunch, I go to the gym.

A typical workout is about one hour of assorted weight-lifting exercises (light weights, high "reps") and three sets of sit-ups. Then I swim a mélange of strokes for about fifteen minutes. Next comes a sauna and shower (a massage once a week) and I go back to the office. I generally work out two times a week (one hour per session) with weights, jog, and do calisthenics (forty-five minutes per session) twice a week and play singles tennis (about one and one-half hours per session) twice weekly.

My weekly work schedule is four days teaching, and I practice for one evening and one-half day on Saturday. In the office, there is a contoured, inclined couch. After the gym session, I usually meditate for about twenty-five minutes while lying on the couch. Then I have a leisurely dinner and endo practice from 6:00 to 9:30. At home, the rest of the evening is for reading, writing and conversation. Sleep usually comes easily and averages about seven and one-half hours.

During the rest of the week, I'm generally home about 5:30. Dinner is with the family, except for about once a week when we "eat out." Evenings are for meetings (about one per week) and relaxation. We frequently go on vacations (average three a year), but I occasionally do some writing and drawing when I'm on a trip. My biggest problem is that I'm a workaholic. I don't like the idea of doing nothing (aside from meditation time and sleep). I like to engage in many pursuits. I've had a few career changes, including microbiology, general dentistry, endodontics, and teaching. And I do have a temper, but my outbursts are infrequent. I like to blame my vicissitudes on my being a Gemini; Dr. Furst says this is pure rationalization — but whatever the case, I enjoy my life. The central theme to my philosophy is to seek and savor life. My parting thought is "enjoy and diversify."

M. F.'s Story

When one considers the fight-or-flight stress response, either course of action can be beneficial physiologically. And although it may be more heroic to fight, it might be more prudent to flee. Part of my coping philosophy is based on this principle. I prefer getting out of the stress situation whenever it is possible; I accomplish this by physical withdrawal or evasion. Generally, I let the Type A's carry the flag and the burden — but I counsel them to bring their compulsive behavior under control.

To counter stressors, I also do other things. For instance, all my life I've engaged in team sports such as basketball. Since 1970, when I discovered running (influenced by Dr. Cooper's book on Aerobics), I run and run and run, and as I run I meditate. I try to run 6 miles every other day, generally starting at 6:30 AM. Actually, I don't like exercise, and running can be boring. But with the conditioning of running, I'm ready to engage in competitive sports during which I'm so busy trying to win that I'm getting the benefits of physical exercise. My favorite sport is tennis (I'm a weekend hacker), and I play four-wall handball or three-man basketball when the occasion arises (at the present time I find them too strenuous.)

Regular periods of meditation are not for me, but I do close out the outside world when a stressful situation threatens. I have my own brand of meditation which I find extremely helpful (an eclectic culling from my experiences with "touching and feeling" encounter groups.) In fact, I've had most of my dental procedures done (since 1970) with a minumum of novocaine, and some major surgery was performed with only a local.

I engage in many diversions; currently, I'm designing a tennis racquet for those who prefer a two-handed forehand as well as backhand. I also make attempts at stained glass windows, picture frames, drawing, and writing. My diet is moving toward a low-fat, low-meat, low-carbohydrate, little sugar and salt, high-fish, vegetable, and salad approach. My staples are yogurt, granola, and fruit.

My parting thought is that I have found that being a tortoise isn't all that bad, if you keep the fate of the hare in mind.

APPENDIX 2

HOW WE DID IT

THE STRESS OF WRITING A BOOK ON STRESS

THE stress of writing a book on stress began before we began. It started when we first had the idea. The first stressor was worry: Who would be the publisher? Would we have the time? How would we write it? Could we work together?

After these issues were resolved, the next job was to structure the book. The ideas came out of the many brainstorming sessions we held. D.M. then used the resources of the health science libraries, while M.F. concentrated his efforts at the main campus library. Relying on their special talents, D.M. undertook outlining and writing the first draft; and M.F. did the rewriting and editing. Fortunately, there were few disagreements as to what belonged where and what should be included in the first place.

Help was sought with the revised first draft. A working copy was perused by friends for their comments and suggestions. Finally, the third and last draft was completed.

For D.M. most of the stress of writing this book was associated with the strain on family relationships. Reading, contemplating, and writing takes an enormous number of hours. The time and pressures involved make it difficult to be a loving husband and an indulgent father. Wife and children were forced to listen to the words of wisdom. This was stressful for at least three reasons. First, most of the time when D.M. wanted them to listen, the family was busy doing something else and really didn't want to be disturbed. Second, when he got them to listen, they disagreed with some of the concepts; hence, there was a major battle or two and several minor skirmishes. Third, the family expected an enlightened husband and father to live up to his words, taking them to fancy restaurants and seeing shows. The defensive response that these things had to be delayed wasn't too well received.

For M.F., most of the stress came from putting on paper what scientists may consider relatively "soft" material, e.g. reports on subjective feelings during stress, hypnosis, and meditation. M.F. felt he could tell others of his experiences as a dental patient, i.e. moving from "I hate dentists" to "I hate going to the dentist" to being grateful for the service they rendered. But, as a psychologist could he inform others via a *book* of how to cope with the stressors of the dental situation?

Another stressful part of creating a book is the waiting. You wait for typing; you wait for the illustrations to be prepared; you wait for the mail; and finally, you wait for that first copy of the published book. There is that special stress that comes in working toward a publication date deadline.

Writing a book is stimulating, but things like indexing can be deadly boring. As we found out, doing the indexing yourself may save some money, but you certainly pay the price. In summation, when all is said and done and the waiting is over, it's all worthwhile.

Other possible sources of stress could have been uncooperative administrators or publishers. The authors were fortunate on both these scores. The department chairmen, the dean, and the publisher, Payne Thomas and his staff, were most helpful throughout the entire process. And finally, although writing any book is stressful, for the authors of this book it definitely was *eustress*.

NAME INDEX

D

E

F

L

M

N

O

P

T

U

V

W

Y

Z

SUBJECT INDEX

G

H

T

U